completely SURRENDER

Suffering By Faith,

My Battle with Depression and Anxiety

HALES

Completely Surrender

Suffering By Faith, My Battle with

Depression and Anxiety

: :

By Makala Wells Hales

: :

Guest Chapters by James M. Hales and Lizza Cazier

Foreword by David Specht

© 2018 Makala W. Hales

: :

Revised Edition: May 2020
No content alterations, only typographical and grammatical corrections.

: :

: :

Medallion design and fabrication by Staci Scheffer of Whackadoodles and Wanderlust (www.whackadoodles.com)

Photography by Rachael Cutler Photo (rachaelcutler.com)

Book formatting design by Joshua Kessie

: :

All Bible references come from the King James Version

: :

ISBN 978-0-9965979-1-3

IF YOU ARE BATTLING

THOUGHTS OF SUICIDE

DON'T WAIT
TO ACT

NATIONAL SUICIDE

PREVENTION LINE

1.800.273.TALK

OR TEXT

741741

TO JAMES, THE HERO

OF MY STORY,

AS WELL AS

MY MOM & DAD, LIZZA,

SHELLY, AND THE BATTALION

OF WOMEN, THEIR HUSBANDS,

AND THEIR FAMILIES WHO

KEPT OUR FAMILY AFLOAT.

C O N T E N T S

FOREWORD

Completely Surrender is the story of Makala Hales, a young mother whose life epitomizes self-reliance, optimism, education and faith in God. A little background may help set the stage for the reader: Makala was a relentless athlete and competitor during her high school years, she lettered in three sports and earned a 4.0 GPA becoming valedictorian. Makala went on to graduate at the top of her nursing class passing her boards only weeks before she began her service as a missionary for her church for 18 months in Ukraine where she learned to fluently speak the Russian language. She returned to work as a nurse in one of the most prominent Neo-Natal units in the country. She achieved each goal she set through the patterns of hard work, discipline and sheer grit that define her character as well as her early married life and becoming a tireless mother of four young children. Then Makala and her husband James were blessed with twins, and for the first time in her life she was confronted with a challenge she could not grind her way through to success. The boys came early and spent time in the hospital gaining their strength. Their birth began a long march that started with miracles and joy, plunged into sleep-deprived sorrow and misery, and made the slow arduous climb back up with more miracles and ultimately, unbelievably, more joy.

Her story is one of courageous independence, unfailing faith and crippling depression and anxiety. Anyone who knows Makala would not believe she could even be susceptible to such dark, lonely and debilitating feelings. It is precisely for that reason I am glad that she is sharing her story. Her story is for the young mother that is struggling with depression. Her story is for the husband that doesn't know how to help his wife. Her story is for the friends and neighbors that notice something is amiss, but don't know how to help. Sadly, her story is the untold story of countless others that are suffering alone, even when surrounded by many willing supporters.

Makala's story is one of spiritual steadiness in her investment to develop a relationship with God and Jesus Christ. Her story highlights the need for each of us to choose to believe in Jesus Christ, put in the work to learn of him and to live like Him and then have the patience to wait and have that faith confirmed.

Completely Surrender is about one woman's desire to candidly tell her story and let it out into the world to help at least one person or family to not have to suffer as she and her family have suffered. This story is brutally personal, not only for the author, but probably for someone that you love. Makala's experience and story became a valuable resource to my family and me as my wife struggled with depression and anxiety following the birth of our youngest child. As a husband, it provided me the understanding and tools I needed to try to be helpful to my wife. Please take time to read her words and take action to relieve suffering and to bring hope to someone around you that may be hurting as she was.

I hope Makala's story will be your inspiration to keep believing. May her story encourage you to more fully access the enabling power of Jesus Christ's Atonement. May her story inspire you to get the help and support you need to heal physically, emotionally, psychologically and spiritually. It is through Christ's suffering that you will find hope to be made whole again. Completely Surrender!!!

—**Dave Specht, author of** *The Family Business Whisperer*

P U R P O S E

I remember where I was, walking alone, the bright-morning sun reflecting heat off the pavement that would give way to a late-summer scorcher day. As I walked, I prayed. I told God, if he would see me to the other side of this black hole, I promised to help anyone with whom I came in contact who suffered likewise. It has been a blessing to keep that promise. I've had the opportunity to connect with those who suffer not only from post-partum depression but also seasonal affective disorder, chronic depression, bipolar disorder, PTSD, and anxiety. Because of what I experienced, I am trusted by those who can sense that I've been where they now are. They have trusted me with their stories, and as a result I have been privileged to "succor the weak, lift up the hands which hang down, and strengthen the feeble knees." (D&C 81:5). When given the opportunity to speak in public settings, I have shared my experience and what it taught me. The response is that those who feel alone, and in the shadows, have expressed their gratitude for my willingness to speak up and speak out. Writing this book is an effort to further keep my promise to God, to help others who suffer as I suffered. At one time in history, a people in bondage were promised by God, "I will...ease the burdens which are put upon your shoulders...that ye may stand as witnesses for me hereafter, and that ye may know of a surety that I, the Lord God, do visit my people in their afflictions" (Mosiah 24:14). This book is my witness "hereafter" of that promise fulfilled for me.

This is meant to be a concise, hopeful message, not a comprehensive, clinical, or exhaustive approach. In the epicenter of depression, exertion to any degree, including reading a self-help book, taxes scarce energy.

It would be wonderful if what I have written here could curb the worst of depression, but I'm guessing if you have searched out a book about depression, you are beyond the first signs and symptoms. If you are reading this, I'm guessing you are now experiencing something over which you feel little control, something dark and overwhelming, something defeating and scary. *I hope that by writing this book, I will validate your experience with my words, and you can find hope and healing*. Depression says, "you are the only one who feels this way, and it's your fault." There is NO truth in that statement. This book is meant to be the friend whose presence is stabilizing, and whose words of encouragement, experience, and promise change the tide, or at least sustain the changing tide, in your journey. I'm going to write this book from me to you, as your friend in the room.

I also realize that one who is suffering from depression, by definition, no longer finds joy in previously enjoyed activities. So, even if you were a "reader" before, I doubt you feel much like engaging in that pursuit right now. And, if you didn't consider yourself a "reader," reading this book is not even something you may have done anyway. With this in mind, I have written this book in short chapters, food for thought, by way of instruction and inspiration, to be digested in small quantities—perhaps while you feed a baby, wait in a doctor's office, or while just sitting with someone who cares. I hope that these small bites will empower you to have just enough "umph" to do just a little at a time and feel more in control of your healing process.

I hope to help those who love the sufferer. Perhaps something here will help you to better understand the "crater" and "dark night of the mind"[1] your loved one is experiencing. There isn't a lot you can do to "fix the problem," but there is a lot you can do to be as Aaron and Hur were to Moses when his "hands were heavy." They "stayed up his hands, the one on the one side, and the other on the other side; and his hands were steady until the going down of the sun" (Exodus 17:12). Just as Israel prevailed when Moses's hands were held up, your loved one will "prevail" as you "stay" and "steady." I have included a chapter written by my husband, James, from his perspective. I have also included a chapter written by an amazing friend, Lizza, who did so much to keep our family afloat while I sunk.

Last but not least, *I hope to help dissolve general misunderstandings and the "hush, hush" nature of depression*. Let me illustrate with an example. My sister, Blaire, recently asked me for advice on how to talk to a friend about post-partum depression. The father of Blaire's friend had suspected his daughter was suffering from depression, but he said to "keep it on the down low." That's the mentality I hope to help dissolve! For some reason (a stigma I will talk about later) people treat depression as a sin, a character flaw, or an unspeakable weakness. As that mentality is fostered, the sufferer not only suffers from depression, but also from feeling shamed. That "hush, hush" mentality is so very unproductive for the sufferer and for those trying to help. I hope to be able to shed light on this condition called depression in such a way as to relieve a significant "hush, hush" factor "that hinders the joy and progress of [man and] woman."[2]

Although I hope this book has the potential to help people of all faiths and walks of life, it is quite obvious that I write it as a faithful member of The Church of Jesus Christ of Latter-day Saints. We believe in a living prophet and apostles who speak the word of God. The words and promises of these living mouthpieces of the Lord were lifelines for me in a very real way. I hope that whether or not you share my faith, the truth of the words of these inspired leaders will speak to your heart and soul as well.

I have been hesitant to write this book, it has been over 7 years since I experienced my plunge into the dark. However, this voice in my mind just keeps saying, "Write the book." I hope you are the one to know why.

PART 1

CRISIS

"His divine love and unfailing help will be with us even when we struggle—no, will be with us especially when we struggle"

(Jeffrey R. Holland, "Tomorrow the Lord Will Do

Wonders among You," Ensign, May 2016).

"...the words of Christ, if we follow their course, [shall] carry us beyond this vale of sorrow into a far better land of promise"

(Alma 37:45).

M Y

S T O R M

CHAPTER 1

✺

In retrospect, it was the perfect storm.

MAY 16, 2011—I waddled into the Parks and Rec Department with my two-year old; I was 7 months pregnant with twins. I had gone to register my kids for summer soccer. We had 9 and 7-year-old sons, and a 5-year-old daughter in addition to the 2-year-old I had in tow. I think I only signed one up for soccer that day; I wasn't being completely unrealistic with twins on the way. It was beautiful springtime, and life was good. I was living my dream of being a young mother with happy, healthy kids.

In the middle of the night, I woke with contractions and by the time we got to the hospital I was too far along to stop the labor. Before 6am on **MAY 17, 2011**, our twin boys were born (the second baby came in a whirlwind emergency C-section)—nearly two months early, at about 4 pounds each. They spent 16 days in the Newborn Intensive Care Unit. Long story short, during that time, I experienced a blood clot and anaphylactic shock including an ambulance ride back to the hospital. While my husband spent the night back in the hospital with me, he went upstairs to visit our baby boys in the NICU. The next few weeks were crazy running back and forth from the hospital to be with babies, juggling the end of the school year for my kids, learning to use a breast pump every three hours, and arranging babysitters for my two little ones still at home during my daily trips to the hospital. My husband was finishing his school year as a teacher and administrator, and in the middle of his Master's Degree.

When our twins were released from the hospital, my mother, my husband, and I spent the rest of the summer dripping milk into the mouths of these tiny boys, constantly on the edge of our chairs for any sign of choking, or cessation of breath. I slept very, very little. As near as I can figure, for three months, I never slept more than 3 consecutive hours and often not more than 3—4 hours total each night.

AUGUST 12, 2011—As much as I had loved sunrises and sunsets all my life, this morning, watching the sun rise broke me. I had always relished the tranquility of early mornings, often running for exercise as the rays broke the horizon, but this sunrise was not welcomed. I had seen sunrise after sunrise over the last few months, not because I was waking to the dawn of a new day, but because I was already awake with feedings and diapers. I couldn't do it anymore. I knelt down by the couch and through tears I told Heavenly Father I just couldn't do it anymore. I had fought the fight, but I was completely spent, plus some. But nothing happened. It was another day.

That night I lay in my bed as my husband read to me and coached me through a muscle relaxation exercise that I had remembered from my college days. My college roommate had experimented on me for one of her classes. She took her time to calmly prompt me to flex and relax each muscle group from my eyebrows to my toes. During the experiment years previous, I had struggled to stay awake—perhaps because of the exercise, perhaps because I am an easy sleeper, quick to sleep, and sleeping deeply until the new day. That night following my husband's prompts was different. I didn't fall sleep, and I felt as though I was shaking, like shivering, but I wasn't cold. I had every reason in the world to be absolutely exhausted. I had single-handedly made it through the night with our infant twins for two nights while my husband was away on business for the first time since they were born. In addition, the first night he was home (the previous night), our four other children had the stomach flu and between the two of us, we managed a night full of twin feedings and many trips to the bathroom with children and their accompanying messes. That sleepless night, in addition to my three months of sleep deprivation, should have been enough to knock me out. I was exhausted, beyond exhausted. But something was wrong, my body was not shutting down for the night.

AUGUST 13, 2011—It was a Saturday morning after another long, sleepless night, that I started to panic knowing how much I needed to sleep, but couldn't. Fully aware of the situation, my mom intervened and insisted my husband take the older kids to a family reunion a couple of hours away, and off they went. A friend of twins came to my rescue and offered to care for my babies so I could take a nap. I went to a back bedroom of our house, away from any noise, and attempted to sleep on my son's bunk bed. My mind started racing with all kinds of fears, mostly of the idea of my children having a "crazy mother." I tried to sleep. My mind spun out of control with irrational thoughts. I prayed, I read the scriptures, I tried to sing hymns, but nothing calmed me. I felt out of control. I was terrified. Looking back, and knowing what I now know, I recognize that nap attempt was a panic attack. (It was a long time before I could lay down on that bed again because my mind had associated that disturbing experience with that particular place.) When I couldn't take it anymore, I went back to the living room where my friend encouraged me to get help and assured me there was help. I felt so desperate; I needed help now.

I called my doctor who was on-call and told her something was wrong. My doctor explained to me that my body was in "fight-or-flight" mode, similar to what would happen if I met a bear in the woods. However, instead of it lasting a few seconds, it would not shut off. I had been so physically, mentally, and emotionally taxed for so long that the chemicals in my brain were depleted, specifically a chemical called serotonin. Decreased levels of serotonin cause anxiety, insomnia, lack of appetite, and depression. She prescribed a medication to help me sleep. For the next couple of weeks I lived in a state of disassociation. I would watch life happen around me but not feel connected to it. I could not "feel" the moments of joy which I knew had made me happy previously. In fact, I could not feel anything. It was as though I was emotionally numb.

By the end of August, I was struggling with my appetite. At first, I just didn't seem to be hungry, but the lack of appetite morphed into just the thought of food completely repulsing me. I force fed myself knowing I had to have fuel for energy to perform my responsibilities with the children. (At that point, these were the terms I was using to refer to the little ones under our roof. "The children," and "the babies," reflect the apathy I felt; I no longer felt connected to the little ones I had carried, given birth to, wept, laughed, and prayed over.) Then I started to vomit. I called the doctor again. When she invited me to look at the list of postpartum depression symptoms, my first thought was, "what I am experiencing is way beyond any emotional 'downer'." Nonetheless, I read them.

- feelings of hopelessness/ helplessness/worthlessness
- social isolation
- anxiety
- "low" feelings and mood
- sleep disturbances
- disturbances of appetite and weight loss/gain
- irritability
- fatigue, loss of energy
- difficulty concentrating
- guilt

My response: "I could have written that list." My doctor diagnosed me with postpartum depression and recommended starting me on an anti-depressant. I have always been one to tough out a headache rather than take a Tylenol, but at that point, I didn't even resist the recommended prescription. She explained that the medication would cause my nervous system to recycle my own serotonin until it could produce serotonin sufficiently on its own. The only problem, the medication would take 4-6 weeks to have full effect. I had a major concern. Each day was an eternity. Each hour was an eternity. I didn't know if I could make it that long.

I became completely dysfunctional. My husband had to take time off work and apply for the Family and Medical Leave Act. My mother spent most of her days helping to take care of the babies and my family. Others came to help.

At that time of year, it was over 100 degrees in the desert climate of southeastern Washington, but I sought out the intense, dry heat which made me feel at least something—hot. Wrought iron legs and arm rests supported the wooden slats of the bench where I would sit in the pea gravel play area of our backyard. I let the blazing sun sear my back through my t-shirt. My elbows were braced on my knees as my hands pressed against my forehead and held the weight of my hanging head. What was happening to me? Why could I feel absolutely nothing but the heat of the sun? What had happened to the person I knew who loved life and people and places?

The blackness I felt was so heavy. A darkness and void set in that I can only describe as "the pains of hell" (Alma 36:13). I knew suicide was wrong, so alternatively, I began to wish I were dead, or at least that someone would knock me out until it was over. Having lived in "the light" my entire life, these feelings were foreign and frightening. I asked the doctor to hospitalize me, but she told me my job was to stay alive by keeping liquids down until the medication kicked in.

My family doctor referred me to a psychiatrist. A few months earlier that would have been unthinkable. In the past, with the limited knowledge and understanding I had had, I would have had a damning hesitancy to go see a psychiatrist. Psychiatrists were for unstable, inept, and "crazy" people. *I was not the type of person that went to a "shrink".* At this point in my depression, the term "psychiatrist," didn't even make me blink. I was so desperate for any kind of help that anyone could offer, and I was willing to take it from anyone who was willing to give it. (Little did I know that an orthopedic specialist is to a torn ACL as a psychiatrist is to a dysfunctional brain.) At that point, I was grateful for the chance at more help, a hoped-for deliverance of some sort.

My psychiatrist changed my sleeping medication to a more restful medication. He also added another medication for severe depression and mood stabilization, and one for panic attacks. Taking serious medications was a new experience for me, and I was anxious about taking such "heavy meds." I knew I really didn't have a choice though, I was on the fast track to destruction if something didn't change quickly.

With reservation, I started taking the medication. I started to feel a difference in my sleep. It started to actually feel like sleep instead of just being "checked-out" for a certain number of hours each night. I went and visited with a therapist who helped me to understand what was going on and what I could do about it. For awhile, I visited both the psychiatrist and the therapist often—one or the other, or both, at least a couple times a week.

Then came the "brain fog" and inability to concentrate accompanied by faulty memory. Conversations were difficult to engage in, simple problem-solving was overwhelming. As is often the case with mental illnesses, my medications and dosages had to be adjusted a few times. Each time brought set-backs and discouragement.

Days came and went ever so slowly — improvement almost imperceptible.

If you can relate to any or all of this, I hope you find the strength to read on and glean from my experience what may help you in yours.

CRISIS

PERIOD

CHAPTER 2

"It is a horrible thing to recognize joy

and not be able to feel it"

(*My journal*, August 26, 2011).

"Sometimes I feel like giving up—in a deep way, not just

the b.t. (before twins) hard days, but hopeless giving up"

(*My journal*, Sept. 1, 2011).

"Most of the time consumed by dark thoughts and the desire for it all to just go away—an endless sleep"

(*My journal*, Sept. 2, 2011).

"Most of today I have been consumed by the feeling that I just want it to end"

(*My journal*, Sept. 3, 2011).

"Everyone says, 'one day at a time.' I don't know if I can keep going. I dread another day"

(*My journal*, Sept 7, 2011)

Unwisely, I passed off the initial cues of postpartum depression to the fact that I had two babies, not one. "Of course, it was going to be more difficult," I told myself. (If you are a member of the "Twins Club," whether you experienced postpartum depression or not, you know that 1+1 does not equal 2. Somehow, two babies feels like 10 babies.) I recognized depression a little late in the game, and rock bottom seemed to come out of nowhere. If you are like me, I won't beat around the bush—you have a long road ahead. I, as well as others, have passed that way before and although it will take more than you feel you have to give, there is much to be learned and gained. Just hold on and keep holding on.

My crisis went something like this. I reached a point where stimulus of nearly every kind was too much for my mind to bear. For what seemed like my very survival, I had to retreat to a dark corner in my bedroom at the back of the house and just sit. After awhile, I couldn't even cry. I couldn't listen to music I knew I liked; I couldn't watch TV; I couldn't handle crowds or even the commotion of family life. Even touch and smells were unpleasant. I could read a little, and I could write a little, and I could pray, and that was about it. I was left to wait out the long hours as close family and friends would come and sit with me. I told them over and over, "I just want out. I just want this to be over." Most devastating, and unexplainable was the fact that I couldn't feel the peace and comfort of the Spirit. The best way I know how to describe it is with J.K. Rowling's description of dementors in *Harry Potter*. In their presence, Harry feels as though the very life is sucked out of him, that every shroud of light is gone, and he is subjected to doom. I called it the Black Hole. That may sound dramatic to anyone who hasn't experienced it, but those who have simply agree.

When depression takes the fast lane to rock bottom, or when left untreated or unaddressed for whatever reason, there is an indescribable period of crisis before medication and/or intervention is effective. The darkness is heavy and the desire to live is absent. Severe depression can lead to what are called "death wishes" as well as suicidal thoughts, or thoughts of harming self, others, or your baby. I now understand the "why" of the shocking stories in the news of mothers who drive themselves and a carload of their children off a bridge. I've been there, I know the despair of their frenzied minds. It doesn't mean they were vile, or evil, or "crazy". It meant they didn't get help before it was too late. Being aware of this reality is crucial. You must also know that those thoughts are not you, but a product of a dysfunctional brain. You must depend upon your knowledge, and not your feelings, that life is valuable and each of our lives is in the hands of the Lord in a very real way. "We affirm the sanctity of life and of its importance in God's eternal plan."[1] Voice your thoughts and fears with those close to you and make sure they take necessary measures to keep you and others safe. For a period of time, I did not trust myself alone. Find, and have on hand, the phone number for a crisis hotline or have someone do it for you. It is a devastating state to be in, but this is one time when it is better to be safe than sorry.

Repeatedly, in my mind's eye at the time, I saw myself dangling off a cliff, my fingers digging into the rock surfaced by sand and loose gravel, ever slipping. I seemed to be dangling constantly, forever grappling. It was desperate, traumatic, scary, and uncharted.

If any of this sounds familiar, I hope you have professional help already on board. If not, the time is NOW! Do not wait any longer to seek out the help that will be the life-preserver for which you are thrashing.

WHEN

MENTAL

FEELS

PHYSICAL

CHAPTER 3

＊

"Could hardly get the liquids down today. So exhausted and weak. Overwhelmed. Felt like I was dying"

(*My journal*, Sept. 6, 2011).

"Today I am grateful for...

not throwing up"

(*My journal*, October 10, 2011).

"exhausted...

exhausted...

exhausted...

exhausted"

(*My journal*, nearly every day).

Even after my initial diagnosis of post-partum depression, I went back and forth to my family doctor, a therapist, a psychiatrist, a naturopath, and a chiropractor. Something felt more wrong than what I understood depression to be. I just kept hoping someone could tell me what was wrong with me. I had blood tests. I had thyroid tests. I had hormone tests. I had genetic tests. I had blood sugar tests. Something just didn't feel right, and I was begging my doctor for more and more tests because I was positive there was something physically wrong with me. My appetite had gone from "not really hungry" to being repulsed by the thought of food, to barely being able to get liquids down only to then vomit. I was losing weight and yet I felt heavy, very heavy, and sluggish. I felt like I was wearing a dentist's lead x-ray shield around all the time. I was completely drained of energy and motivation. Physically, it felt like the flu with no relief. Mentally, I felt foggy and dull.

"Mental" does not mean "mental" in the way it is generally stigmatized. "Mental" simply means there is something physically wrong with your central nervous system, primarily the chemicals in your brain. These chemicals called neurotransmitters (you may have heard of serotonin, dopamine, or norepinephrine—three of the identified neurotransmitters) are substances that travel from the end of one nerve to the next nerve to transfer impulses. They play the role of communication in the vast complexity of our nervous system and brain. Their proper adequacy and balance are imperative for not only our well-being, but also our sense of well-being. Included in the list of those aspects of our lives which these neurotransmitters regulate are things we typically categorize as both physical and mental: appetite, sleep, logical thinking and problem-solving, sense of well-being, levels of interest, feelings of self-worth and confidence, just to summarize. When the neurotransmitters are insufficient or out of balance, we feel broken; we feel something is wrong.

Unlike more obvious set-backs of our physical body, whether broken or diseased, depression is not something that can be easily seen with our eyes. In fact, there is very little in the medical field to objectively test for depression—no blood tests, no CAT scans or MRIs, no x-rays. Because of that, depression has been misunderstood for centuries because it cannot be seen or measured.

The chemical insufficiency or imbalance can be the result of a plethora of causes. Some people may be genetically predisposed as our chemical make-up comes from the same DNA which dictates hair color and height, as well as tendencies to heart disease or diabetes. Others may experience a long draw of stress on their chemical resources depleting their levels. Major life changes also take a toll on our chemical stores and balances.

So, don't be quick to doubt a "mental illness" diagnosis from a healthcare professional if you are feeling something is physically wrong. It is. It is physically wrong in your brain and so it is termed, "mental illness."

A N X I E T Y

CHAPTER 4

✴

"I woke up anxious...just enough to make me uncomfortable and disconnected from what's going on around me—and to guide my thoughts irrationally"

(*My journal*, August 22, 2011).

"Anxiety makes it so I feel numb, distanced from reality, simply going through the motions. It is what I know right now that I'm trusting in. Not what I feel—because it is so hard to feel anything positive"

(*My journal*, September 1, 2011).

"Battled anxiety most of the day.."

(*My journal*, Oct. 13, 2011).

"My storm" started with anxiety. I had had "butterflies" plenty of times in my life. As a sophomore in high school, I would even get so nervous on the days of my World History tests that I would get sick to my stomach and couldn't eat breakfast. We all have anxieties in life that give us that nervous feeling—a blind date, a public presentation, a final exam. Those anxieties come and go with the experiences with which they are associated. The anxiety we are talking about here, either independently or associated with depression, is different. It builds and builds with no release. It becomes paralyzing.

When my doctor explained my anxiety to me, she talked about the "fight or flight response." This is part of the autonomic nervous system—that innate system within us that governs all of our amazing functions that we don't conscientiously control, such as heart rate, blood pressure and digestion. The autonomic nervous system has two parts: the sympathetic and parasympathetic divisions. The sympathetic system, "fight or flight," kicks in when we are under stress—heart rate and blood pressure shoot up, breathing accelerates and digestion grinds to a halt. This is a great design when we are truly in peril—it ups our game, and puts all non-essential systems on stand-by. When true danger has passed, the parasympathetic system engages and turns off the stress response returning heart rate, breathing and blood pressure to normal. The parasympathetic system is referred to as the "rest and digest" system. When the big game, test or presentation is over, this is the system in action when we feel a great sense of relief and feel at ease again, perhaps we feel like a big meal and a nap. However, when the brain irrationally sends a constant message of danger, the sympathetic nervous system cycles the response and the message back and forth until full-blown panic occurs. The body actually doesn't know the difference between the thought of threat and actual threat itself. If a message of threat is sent by the brain, the body reacts as though it is actually in danger. When that "feeling" of danger registers in our brain it reinforces the thought of threat so the brain resends the threat message again. The sympathetic nervous systems overpowers the parasympathetic nervous system and the result is prolonged and intensifying anxiety. The good news is that the brain is magnificent enough that with conscious effort it can stimulate the parasympathetic nervous system through thought. This is where interventions such as cognitive behavioral therapy and yoga come in—they train you to force your thoughts to stimulate "rest and digest" over "fight or flight." This is why we "feel" certain emotions as we remember, or even imagine, certain events. Our body is responding to a thought.

With my anxiety, the predominant feeling I experienced was that I was on the edge of breakdown. It felt as though any additional stressor would put me over the edge. I was only one knock on the door, one phone call, or one crying child away from being done for. That is the feeling of "fight or flight." I didn't feel I had it in me to either fight or fly. That feeling makes a person want to crawl into a ball and keep everything out.

When I was eventually diagnosed with post-partum depression, it seemed like the paradox of paradoxes. I was supposed to be "depressed," but yet so often I felt like crawling out of my skin. "Depressed" was supposed to be "low," and yet I was so "anxed up" I felt jittery. ("Anx" isn't a dictionary word, it's my own verb for the noun "anxiety.") It was news to me that anxiety is a very common symptom of depression.

Defined, anxiety means, "distress or uneasiness of mind caused by fear of danger or misfortune" (dictionary.com). As I experienced my own anxiety, and as I have had several experiences with others and their anxiety, it seems that the mind wraps around a specific concern—a person, an event (past or feared), a condition—a dread of one kind or another. It is like an electrician who unknowingly grasps a charged wire and the electrical current stimulates the muscles to forcefully contract such that it is impossible to let go. For some reason, it is the same with the mind. The mind wraps around this "wire" and won't let go. The longer and the firmer the mind wraps around the "wire" the more irrational and extreme the thoughts become. For the electrician, death from electrocution comes unless the electrician is physically hit by force to separate the hand from the wire. With anxiety associated with depression, serious alterations to life result—can't sleep, can't eat, can't concentrate, can't drive... Some kind of "hit" has to take place to restore balance.

Anxiety is, at the very least, distracting from normal activity. Most often, it causes sleep disturbances which quickly wear a person thin. At worst, it is debilitating. When anxiety begins to disrupt life for more than a short period of time, then is the time that the interventions for anxiety and depression must take place in order for the brain chemistry to heal and rebalance, and for your well-being to be restored. These interventions are varied. These interventions may or may not include medication, and they will be discussed later in this book.

If the anxiety isn't addressed, it seems to dig a rut in the mind—deeper and deeper. The deeper the rut, the more difficult to get out of it. It is definitely to your advantage to not try and fight it alone, but to be open about it, and get help sooner than later.

I found myself trying to determine if the anxiety I felt was caused by my chemical imbalance, or if it was caused by what I was thinking about or doing. That seemingly ever-present battle was always fruitless, there is no way to find that fine tip black line in all the gray. I wanted to be able to control as much as I could control, but the reality was, I never knew where "my thinking" stopped and where the chemical imbalance began.

The best approach I found is captured well in a BYU Magazine article by Erin Holmes. She speaks of anxieties in general and references BYU Professor, Gregory Clark's 2008 Devotional address.

"Clark argued that when we wake up every day, we choose to be either faithful or fearful. When we choose faith, we minimize fear. When we choose fear, hope and faith are virtually impossible. He explained: 'When I am living in fear, I find change and changing—for the better, at least—almost impossible. It is important to learn how to live in faith rather than fear because the process of changing for the better is at the very foundation of the Father's plan for us.' He then asked, 'What is the source of fear?' I really like his answer: 'I think it is rooted in the assumption....that I must solve all my problems and face all my challenges alone, using my own resources. That is frightening, because deep in my heart I know how limited those resources are....Knowing that I am not capable of changing myself or my circumstances for the better, I stand frozen in fear.' Fear comes from the false belief that we are all alone. What then is the source of faith and hope? Professor Clark said, 'Faith is founded upon our memory of divine witnesses and blessings received in the past and upon our hope in divine promises for the future.'"[1] (I will talk about journaling and the "memory of divine witnesses" in a later chapter.)

Just waking up and choosing faith doesn't "just happen" when chemical anxiety is at play, but the principle applies. We are better off to not fight the battle of "what is chemical and what is me?" Adhere to medical counsel and then just keep choosing faith, faithful thinking. That is battle enough!

INFALLIBLE TRUTH, YOU ARE LOVED

CHAPTER 5

✳

"H. chose to sing "I Am A Child of God"

for FHE. It was as sweet as it gets"

(*My journal*, Oct. 17, 2011)

The definition of "infallible" drives home the gravity of this chapter. Infallible is defined as:

1. absolutely trustworthy or sure

2. unfailing in effectiveness or operation; certain[1]

What was true before *is still true*.

Right now, you might feel that there is nothing about you worthy of being loved. That thought is the voice of depression; it simply is not true. Here begins the task of trusting in what you know, and not what you feel. We are taught, and we learn by faith and experience, to trust the Spirit— those feelings and impressions that come to us. The feelings you have when suffering from depression are not from the Spirit. When the voice of depression tells you that you are worthless, unlovable, and hopeless, you can know that is not a voice to trust. "Remember, our Savior, Jesus Christ, always builds us up and never tears us down".[2] Trusting what you know, and not listening to what you feel (the voice of depression), may seem contrary to the pattern which you have developed. For a time, you will need to trust in what you know and not what you feel.

> The truth is in a prophet's voice, "...your Heavenly Father loves you— each of you. That love never changes. It is not influenced by your appearance, by your possessions, or by the amount of money you have in your bank account. It is not changed by your talents and abilities. It is simply there. It is there for you when you are sad or happy, discouraged or hopeful. God's love is there for you whether or not you feel you deserve love. It is simply always there."[3]

> Alexandre Dumas's words ring true:

> "Abbe Faria: Here is your final lesson – do not commit the crime for which you now serve the sentence. God said, Vengeance is mine.

Edmond Dantes: I don't believe in God.

Abbe Faria: It doesn't matter. **He believes in you.**"[4]

From the get-go, the most significant thing I can say is that I testify to you that Heavenly Father and Jesus Christ know you. They love you. Despite how far away they may feel to you in your life right now, they are NOT far. In fact, as you struggle, they are closer than ever, whether you feel that or not. I echo the Apostle Paul's words and testimony, another individual who experienced severe mortal challenges. He said that God is not an unknown God, and you are not unknown to God, but that "...he [God] be not far from any one of us" (Acts 17:27). *He be not far from any one of us.* Let that thought bring power to your down-trodden spirit.

I love Psalms 147:4, "He telleth the number of the stars; *he calleth them all by their names*" (emphasis added). If you have ever wondered at the night heavens as I have, this verse reminds us that if God knows all the names of all those formations of elements, surely he knows your name, His very offspring.

Comforting is Enoch's observation just after he saw in vision the vast expanses of God's creations, "And were it possible that man could number the particles of the earth, yea, millions of earths like this, it would not be a beginning to the number of thy creations; and thy curtains are stretched out still; *and yet thou art there, and thy bosom is there...*" (Moses 7:30, emphasis added). To me, Enoch's observation is that despite the mind-reeling endlessness of all our Heavenly Father has created, He is there, right there, and His bosom, His heart, is right there. His heart is right there in the center of your life, in the center of your suffering.

I know how hard it is to feel that love, perhaps impossible. However, no matter how difficult it is for you to feel the spirit of peace and love right now in your life, it is my prayer that somehow you can feel God's love through my testimony. It is my prayer that you can know **God's love** *for you is real*, and that **you are not left on your own** during this time. It is an unfailing, certain, even infallible truth—you are loved. What was true before **is still true**.

THE

PLAGUE

CHAPTER 6

☀

"Today I talked to Carrie's sister, Amy who had

post-partum depression + twins. I have talked to

a lot of people who have survived post-partum

depression, but not post-partum depression + twins"

(*My journal*, Oct 28, 2011)

The world has known many plagues since its beginning. The plagues of Egypt, the Bubonic Plague, and smallpox epidemics are among the many plagues with very visible and disastrous effects. Depression is one of the plagues of our day. Depression, unlike the plagues of Egypt, the Bubonic Plague, and smallpox epidemics, encroaches quietly and doesn't express itself with boils, or fevers, or blisters. Depression, like the other plagues, has disastrous effects—it is painful, debilitating, and widespread. I mention this because you probably feel as though you are isolated in your suffering. One of the most surprising things to me was to learn how many people I knew who suffer or have suffered from depression, or who have close family or friends who suffer. It is estimated that one in four people will suffer from depression at some time in their life. It isn't just the numbers of people who suffer that surprised me, but also it is **who** the people are. Amazing people. Amazing people suffer from depression. No one is immune to depression. The talented, the wealthy, the successful, the humble, the righteous, the optimist, male and female, young and old— all are susceptible. There is no inoculation or immunization.

1st Corinthians 10:13 states, "There hath no temptation taken you but such as is common to man..." This scripture speaks of temptation, but I have thought of it over and over again as I learn about yet another person who faces depression. The struggle with depression is common to man, and to woman. It just is. You need not feel isolated in your experience. If we substitute "suffer" for "tempt," I feel the balance of the scripture holds true, "but God is faithful, who will not suffer you to *suffer* above that ye are able; but will with the *suffering* also make a way to escape, that ye may be able to bear it." I know that to be true, absolutely true. The "escape," the "cure" in terms of plagues, has everything to do with the Savior, his perfect empathy, and his enabling power.

PART 2

HOPE

"When we are in darkness, we are more likely to lose hope because we cannot see the peace and joy that await us if we just keep pressing forward"

(Dieter F. Uchtdorf, "Bearers of Heavenly Light," *Ensign*, Nov. 2017, pg. 78).

"Faith in Christ is the only thing to

save you from despair"

(C.S. Lewis, *Joyful Christian.* 1977).

"Believe in miracles. I have seen so many of

them come when every other indication would

say that hope was lost. Hope is never lost"

(Jeffrey R. Holland, "Like a Broken Vessel," *Ensign*, Nov. 2013).

"...hope we have as an anchor of the

soul, both sure and steadfast..."

(Hebrews 6:19).

"There may be times when we must make

a courageous decision to hope even when

everything around us contradicts this hope"

(Dieter F. Uchtdorf, "The Infinite Power of Hope," *Ensign*, Nov. 2008.)

DEPRESSION AND THE ATONEMENT OF JESUS CHRIST

CHAPTER 7

✸

"He wants to heal us, and some wounds can only be healed through the power of the Atonement of Jesus Christ. How? I don't know. But, I know it's true. "O how great the goodness of our God, who prepareth a way for our escape from the grasp of this awful monster... (2 Nephi 9:10)"

. (*My journal*, September 23, 2011)

"As we remember Him and trust in His power,

we receive strength through His Atonement. It

is the means whereby we can be relieved of our

anxieties, our burdens, and our suffering"

(*My journal*, Oct. 13, 2011, quoting Carl B. Cook from

October General Conference 2011).[1]

The idiom, "last but not least" comes to mind as I write this chapter. "Last" because I have written all the other chapters prior to writing this one, "but not least" because this chapter is the greatest key to hope and healing. This chapter is the last to be written because it is the most difficult to write. In Tad Callister's words, "certain thoughts of the spirit are so lofty, so poignant, that they cannot be reduced to the oral language or written word of man."[2] I simply cannot find words to explain or describe how my experience brought me to know Jesus Christ and the power of His Atonement in my life. What was once a horrific time of my life, I now describe as hallowed. When we learn intimately of things beyond this world, this world's words don't fit. "We feel much more than we can tell."[3]

That being said, I fail in the underpinnings of this whole effort to write a book if I don't somehow help you to access the same experience on your own terms. This chapter, though last written, is found in the beginning of this undertaking because it is foundational to the development and success of anything else I might say.

As multi-faceted and deep as the Atonement of Jesus Christ is, there are three most prominent things I learned, or came to more fully appreciate, through my experience. These are: the **comfort** that comes from knowing there is One who perfectly understands, the reality of the **enabling power** of the Atonement of Jesus Christ, and the literal *healing* that takes place by the power of the Atonement of Jesus Christ.

One priceless aspect of the Atonement of Jesus Christ is the knowledge that someone knows exactly how *I* feel, someone knows exactly how *you* feel. This is not blanket coverage, but as individual and personal as my own unique existence, and your unique existence.

Paul taught this truth, "Wherefore in all things it behoved him to be made like unto his brethren" (Hebrews 2:16-17). "All things" definitely embraces what you are experiencing.

An equally reassuring thought is that the Savior is, "touched with the feeling of our infirmities" (Hebrews 4:15). He is touched by what we are going through, not in a sympathetic way, but in an empathetic way. He has been there.

Alma describes the Savior's perfect empathy in detail, "And he shall go forth, suffering pains and afflictions and temptations of every kind; and this that the word might be fulfilled which saith he will take upon him the pains and the sicknesses of his people. ... and he will take upon him their infirmities, that his bowels may be filled with mercy, according to the flesh, that he may know according to the flesh how to succor his people according to their infirmities" (Alma 7:11-12). Although inaccurate, when we suffer from depression, we feel as though no one could possibly understand what it really feels like. To know that the Savior absolutely and perfectly knows is a priceless comfort.

Another valuable lesson I came away with from my experience is that there is a very real enabling power of the Atonement of Jesus Christ. Carolyn Rasmus explained this reality well in her March 2013 Ensign article:

David A. Bednar of the Quorum of the Twelve Apostles said, "I suspect that [we] are much more familiar with the nature of the redeeming power of the Atonement than we are with the enabling power of the Atonement."

He suggested that most of us understand that Christ came to earth to die for us, to pay the price for our sins, to make us clean, to redeem us from our fallen state, and to enable every person to be resurrected from the dead.

But, Elder Bednar said, "I frankly do not think many of us 'get it' concerning [the] enabling and strengthening aspect of the Atonement, and I wonder if we mistakenly believe we must make the journey from good to better and become a saint all by ourselves through sheer grit, willpower, and discipline, and with our obviously limited capacities."

The belief that through our own "sheer grit, willpower, and discipline" we can manage just about anything seems to be widespread these days. This simply is not true.

Heavenly Father and the Savior can inspire, comfort, and strengthen us in our time of need, if we remember to cast our burdens at Their feet.[4]

"Hard" is redefined when struggling with depression. I had done some "hard" things in life. I had grown up on a farm and learned to physically work hard. I participated in three sports a year in high school and learned how to compete hard. I finished a rigorous Nursing Program while working part-time and learned to study hard. I served a foreign mission in Ukraine and learned to endure hard and pray hard. I had done some very demanding things that stretched me physically and mentally, not the least of which was mothering small children with good mental health. However, I had never come close to this new "hard". It isn't something that I think can be described in words—only experienced. I had dug down pretty deep in several of my life's goals and pursuits, but I had never had to dig down as deep as I did to fight my way out of depression. It was the enabling power of the Atonement of Jesus Christ that made up for my deficiencies after, *and while*, all I could do, and gave me the strength to do things that were beyond my own capacity.

I remember distinctly the words coming to me as I trudged through one day, "I'll strengthen thee, help thee, and cause thee to stand, upheld by my righteous, omnipotent hand." When I looked up the hymn, I knew it's author must have had to dig deep at some point to pen words so perfect.

How Firm A Foundation

In ev'ry condition—in sickness, in health,

In poverty's vale or abounding in wealth,

At home or abroad, on the land or the sea—

As thy days may demand, so thy succor shall be.

Fear not, I am with thee; oh, be not dismayed,

For I am thy God and will still give thee aid.

I'll strengthen thee, help thee, and cause thee to stand,

Upheld by my righteous...omnipotent hand.

When through the deep waters I call thee to go,

The rivers of sorrow shall not thee o'erflow,

For I will be with thee, thy troubles to bless,

And sanctify to thee...thy deepest distress.

When through fiery trials thy pathway shall lie,

My grace, all sufficient, shall be thy supply.

The flame shall not hurt thee; I only design

Thy dross to consume...and thy gold to refine.

The soul that on Jesus hath leaned for repose

I will not, I cannot, desert to his foes;

That soul, though all hell should endeavor to shake,

I'll never, no never, I'll never, no never,

I'll never, no never, no never forsake![5]

Alma described tapping into the enabling power of Christ's atoning sacrifice, "...in his strength I can do all things..." (Alma 26:25) as did Paul, "I can do all things through Christ which strengtheneth me" (Philippians 4:13). The enabling power of the Atonement of Jesus Christ has been available for centuries, and it is available to you.

True, real healing is the other aspect of the Atonement I came to know. We understand that the Savior redeems us from our sins when we repent by "remembering them no more." (D&C 58:42). It is as if our slate is wiped clean in His eyes. Interesting to me is another definition of the word "redeem." It means, "make up for; make amends for; offset."[6] One of my greatest fears was that I had lost me, that I would never be whole again. I felt wounded, deeply. This is my journal entry just near the beginning of my ordeal:

I just got off the phone with my sister, Taneil. As we spoke of my experience over the last few days she testified to me that because of the power of the Atonement I will be the same again. Then she said, "No, you will never be the same, you will be the better for it." She said because of the Atonement this condition can be completely healed with time. I felt that assurance. After hanging up, I knelt and thanked Heavenly Father for the Atonement as I have never been grateful before. I pled that through the mercy and the power of the Atonement, the balm of the Atonement will heal me mentally and physically. I know that it will, and that I will be a better wife and mother for it." (*My journal*, August 17, 2011).

It got much worse before it got better, and there were months of deep depression following that conversation, but I can say that she was right. Even after the crisis period had passed, and the "wounds" were no longer fresh and painful, there were still things left "undone," so to speak. I continued to pray for healing, for me and for my family, for months and months and months. That healing has come. Those things that seem lost can be made up for and offset by the Atonement of Jesus Christ—true, real healing. I've dedicated a chapter later in the book just to this subject. Suffice it to say here that the healing power of the Atonement of Jesus Christ is evident and undeniable in my life.

In my mind, as I try to relate my experience to what I now know and feel about the Atonement of Jesus Christ, a question comes: How is it that the very thing we would not wish upon anyone, is the same thing we wouldn't trade for the world? It is because in our extremities we come to know Him—if, we choose it to be so.

S T I G M A

CHAPTER 8

✴

The word "stigma" means a "mark of disgrace or infamy; a stain or reproach, as on one's reputation."[1] Sadly, depression carries with it a definite stigma. Instead of treating depression as an illness or injury, society treats depression as a sin or a character defect. This stigma causes those who suffer to be shameful and secretive. Those who are close to the sufferer, lacking correct understanding, can unknowingly reinforce that shame and secrecy. This lack of understanding and approach do not bless the life of the sufferer.

"The world has a long history of rejecting that which it does not understand. And it has particular trouble understanding things it cannot see."[2] Although science has made great strides in understanding depression, because depression is still difficult to understand, the stigma remains. Also, because depression is difficult to understand, it has been, and is marked in society by shame. I, myself, have been tempted to think less of someone known to struggle with depression, as if they were weak, as if it were their choice. Elder Holland has said, "there should be no more shame in acknowledging them [mental illnesses or emotional disorders] than in acknowledging a battle with high blood pressure or the sudden appearance of a malignant tumor."[3]

You might be surprised to know that some of the grandest accomplishments in this world are attributed to those who have at times struggled with depression, not the least of which are Joseph and Emma Smith, Winston Churchill, and Abraham Lincoln.

Depression is NEITHER a character defect, a bad attitude, a lack of willpower, a weakness, insufficient effort, a sin, nor a punishment. The illness we call "depression" is the state of lessened activity and strength of the chemical activity of the brain and central nervous system. The term comes from the meaning of the root "depress" which means "to lessen the activity or strength of."[4]

Thus, the illness of lessened strength and activity of the brain chemicals was termed "depression." We as humans have then attached all kinds of incorrect and misleading meanings, including all those that depression is NOT.

Even with an accurate understanding of what depression is, it can still be a shameful confession because of what everybody else thinks depression is. When tempted to be shamed, you may want to think of this:

When I looked up the word "stigma" in the dictionary there was another definition. It was as surprising as it was powerful, and I believe it to be a much better association with the battle of depression. It read, "bodily wounds or pains resembling the wounds of the crucified Christ."[5] I read it over, and over again. "Bodily wounds or pains resembling the wounds of the crucified Christ." As I reflect on those darkest days of my life, I recognize that my experience opened a window to my spiritual eyes and gave me a deeper understanding of what happened in the Garden of Gethsemane. The suffering that consumed me was a very minuscule drop in the cup the Savior drank that night. Why? Why would He do that?

Why would the Father let his Only Begotten suffer so? Love. A love which knows no bounds and which hasn't changed. A love so powerful that even if you were the only one ever to walk this earth, The Father and the Son would have done the exact same thing...for you. The "stigma," the bodily wounds and pains of depression sufficiently resemble the wounds of the crucified Christ as to give us a much deeper understanding of His love for us.

HALES

TENDER MERCIES

CHAPTER 9

✦

"For a short while at dinner time I was able

to eat and somehow I could feel life again.

Lizza says it was a tender mercy"

(*My journal*, Nov. 8, 2011).

Elder Bednar teaches the reality and beauty of tender mercies:

> We should not underestimate or overlook the power of the Lord's tender mercies. The simpleness, the sweetness, and the constancy of the tender mercies of the Lord will do much to fortify and protect us in the troubled times...When words cannot provide the solace we need or express the joy we feel, when it is simply futile to attempt to explain that which is unexplainable, when logic and reason cannot yield adequate understanding about the injustices and inequities of life, when mortal experience and evaluation are insufficient to produce a desired outcome, and when it seems that perhaps we are so totally alone, truly we are blessed by the tender mercies of the Lord and made mighty even unto the power of deliverance (see 1 Ne. 1:20).[1]

On many occasions, when it seemed as though I couldn't make it to the surface for one more breath of air, when being swallowed up seemed inevitable, God's tender mercies delivered the rescue needed for the moment. I will recount one example which shows just how mindful God is of each of us, how He knows who to send to the rescue, and how He works in mysterious ways.

Deep into the gloom, a great friend and former college roommate who lived a couple states away, called me one day having heard of my struggles. Although feeling ashamed, I filled in the blanks of what she had heard. She told me she had a good friend, Shelly, who had experienced something she thought sounded very much the same, and asked if it would be all right if Shelly called me. I agreed, very much hoping for answers and direction.

Shortly thereafter, I was sitting, heavy and hollow, on my couch at home waiting for the years to tick away on the clock before my first appointment with the psychiatrist when Shelly called. She introduced herself, and then one of the first things Shelly said to me was, "I can tell by your voice that you are where I have been." My voice had lost all expression, intonation, and emotion. It was completely deflated and flat, just like my soul. We went on to have a conversation in which she described to me what I was experiencing from her own experience, seven years prior. She told me about her process of healing, including professional help, and her witness that God saw her through her hell and He would see me through mine. Somewhere in the conversation, with love and emphasis she said, "Never Surrender." With a glimpse of light at the end of the tunnel, miraculously, when I ended the phone call, I was able to eat an apple, something I had not been able to do for over a week. That afternoon, my husband took me to see the psychiatrist for the first time.

Her words, "Never Surrender," became my bulwark in the following months as I repeated them to myself and she shepherded me at every hour of the day, through texts and phone calls, through all the ups and downs of healing. Shelly's voice became the sound of peace and comfort imperative in my moments of extremity.

A friend followed a prompting and a loving Heavenly Father connected me to my lifeline over a thousand miles away, someone I had never met.

A year later, appropriately for the twins' first birthday, we threw a "survivor" party, complete with tiki torches. We invited all who had been so instrumental in helping us "survive" the previous 12 months. Shelly, and my friend who followed the prompting, surprised us at that party, and I met Shelly face-to-face for the first time. I am guessing, seeing and hugging Shelly for the first time, is as close as I will get in this life to an experience that resembles meeting my Savior in the life to come. Words fail.

There were many, many other tender mercies on my journey. Receiving tender mercies requires an open heart, an open mind, and often an open door.

T R I A L   O F   F A I T H

CHAPTER 10

☀

"This morning before church I thought I was going

to go crazy—just that out of control feeling...I bore

my testimony that it has been the experience of

my life that God has always kept his promises

and it is my faith that he will continue to do so"

(*My journal*, Sept. 2, 2011).

"[I] read in The Friend [magazine] to Sariah this afternoon: 'To have true faith you must trust in the Lord's will and His timing. – Elder Oaks'"

(*My journal*, October 16, 2011).

The depth of the darkness and a frenzied mind, combined with the absence of peace, fathered a soul-searching question for me. It was my understanding that a person sincerely trying to adhere to the gospel of Jesus Christ would never be left to feel the way I felt. Reasoning would mean that either I was not in harmony with the gospel, *OR* the promises were not true. One, or the other. Although not nearly perfect, I knew there was not a transgression in my life which warranted the void of the Spirit I was experiencing. That reason did not apply. And so, the question, "Are the promises true?" The words I had heard nearly every Sunday in my life lingered in my thoughts, "and keep his commandments which he hath given them, that they may always have his Spirit to be with them" (Moroni 4:3). "Always" included now, and I could not feel the Spirit with me now. All my reasoning seemed to conclude that the promise is not valid.

Elder Holland refers to depression as "a crater in the mind" and a "dark night of the mind."[1] That description is very telling. Depression for me was a darkness, a void, an abandonment, a flatness, a gloom that I didn't know existed. The feelings of the spirit which had been prevalent in my life—light, warmth, comfort, and peace—were beyond my reach. No matter how I tried, those longed-for feelings stayed beyond my grasp. I didn't know, and was frankly shocked, that this could happen to a member of the church who was trying to live the principles of the gospel. The result was that I was faced with a very poignant trial of my faith. Would I continue to keep my covenants OR would I harden my heart against a God who I felt had abandoned me and His promises? A wise friend who had experienced a similar trial of her faith wisely counseled me, "what was true before *is still true*." And so I chose to do my best to continue to keep my covenants with the hope, often minuscule, that I wouldn't be subject to the effects of depression forever.

Gratefully, I had had many experiences in my life which testified of God's reality, many of which were beyond reason. I knew God's ways were not my ways, and His thoughts were not my thoughts (Isaiah 55:8-9). I chose to trust. I chose to keep turning to Him. I chose not to turn my back in accordance with my reason, but rather to press forward, one heavy step at a time, searching for the hope of a brighter day. I felt much like Paul's words to the Romans describing Father Abraham's faith when promised seed from "his own body now dead" and "the deadness of Sara's womb... *who against hope believed in hope*" (Romans 4:18-19, italics added). *I did not feel hope, but I believed in hope. That belief was a choice.*

Mostly in retrospect, I can see now how God kept his promise. When I could not feel the Spirit myself, I was almost constantly surrounded by those who carried the Spirit with them in their service and love. In a very real way, God kept his promise to "always have his Spirit to be with [me]" (Moroni 4:3). "With me" was not something felt inside of me as I was accustomed to the fulfillment of that promise, but "with me" in my home, in my life, in my struggles were others who had The Spirit with them.

Speaking of covenants, Elder Christofferson has said, "In these divine agreements, God binds himself to sustain, sanctify, and exalt us in return for our commitment to serve Him and keep His commandments."[2] The scriptures are the written record of these promises kept repeatedly over the centuries...unequivocally. I add my testimony to that of the prophets. "But the Lord knoweth all things from the beginning; wherefore, he prepareth a way to accomplish all his works among the children of men; for behold, he hath all power unto the fulfilling of all his words. And thus it is. Amen" (1 Nephi 9:6).

I absolutely love Michael McLean's father's thought:

Isn't it interesting that the Greatest Intelligence in the Universe abandoned His Son at the most pivotal moment in His plan? Could it be that it was at this moment that the Greatest Intelligence of All bore witness to the universe that He had put His faith in Jesus? That He knew Jesus would choose Him no matter what? And could it be that when you think He has abandoned you that He is actually saying, "I have faith you will choose me even when I'm not there?"[3]

When we face a crisis of our faith, when we feel abandoned, it is by using our agency to choose God that our faith grows. Does that thought not perfectly coincide with the doctrine that all we truly possess to give to God is our own will? When we are completely void of His presence, even of his promised Spirit, that is the moment, (perhaps the many, many long moments) when we are faced with the same choice—to act in faith and choose God, to give Him our will. The alternative is to retain our will in favor of our doubts, choosing to believe that if "I can't feel You, You aren't there." As you meet your trial of faith head on, God is trusting you to choose Him.

In a message entitled, "Trial of Your Faith," Elder Anderson related the following:

> The Apostle Peter identified something he called a "trial of your faith." He had experienced it. Remember Jesus's words:
>
> "Simon, … Satan hath desired to have you, that he may sift you as wheat: But I have prayed for thee, that thy faith fail not."
>
> Peter later encouraged others: "Think it not strange," he said, "concerning the fiery trial which is to try you, as though some strange thing happened unto you."

These fiery trials are designed to make you stronger, but they have the potential to diminish or even destroy your trust in the Son of God and to weaken your resolve to keep your promises to Him…

How do you remain "steadfast and immovable" during a trial of faith? You immerse yourself in the very things that helped build your core of faith: you exercise faith in Christ, you pray, you ponder the scriptures, you repent, you keep the commandments, and you serve others.

When faced with a trial of faith—whatever you do, you don't step away from the Church! Distancing yourself from the kingdom of God during a trial of faith is like leaving the safety of a secure storm cellar just as the tornado comes into view.[4]

When we are confronted with a trial of our faith we have our agency to choose our response to it. The Nephites, when faced with years of war, loss, and destruction encountered the same decision: "because of the exceedingly great length of the war between the Nephites and the Lamanites *many had become hardened*, because of the exceedingly great length of the war; and *many were softened* because of their affliction, insomuch that they did humble themselves before God, even in the depth of humility" (Alma 62:41). Same circumstances, different response. Choose to be the softened clay in the Master's hand. Allow him to teach and mold you through this challenge into someone better than you could be without it. As Elder Hallstrom has lovingly counseled, "Never let an earthly circumstance disable you spiritually."[5]

While on my mission, I read one of Elder Holland's messages quoting President George Q. Cannon in Conference. The words were so inspirational and influential to me then that I put them to memory. Although my mind was foggy during my depression, it remembered these words, and I repeated them to myself regularly:

No matter how serious the trial, how deep the distress, how great the affliction, [God] will never desert us. He never has, and He never will. He cannot do it. It is not His character [to do so]...We may pass through the fiery furnace; we may pass through deep waters; but we shall not be consumed nor overwhelmed. We shall emerge from all these trials and difficulties the better and purer for them, if we only trust in our God and keep His commandments.[6]

You shall emerge from the depths of depression the better and the purer for it, if you only trust in your God and keep His commandments.

"Let us hold fast the profession of our faith without wavering; (for he is faithful that promised;)" (Hebrews 10:23).

OBEDIENCE BRINGS THE BLESSINGS OF HEAVEN

CHAPTER 11

✹

"Laid in bed for probably an hour after I woke this morning. Couldn't bear the thought of facing another day like yesterday. Finally, James came in and I got up for scriptures"

(*My journal*, Nov. 11, 2011).

As a missionary, I knew that if I was following the little white handbook completely, every slammed door or cold shoulder was the result of another's agency, and not God's lack of favor because of my personal failings. This brought a great deal of comfort and peace to me as a missionary. The same principle really applies to every season of our lives. When we are right with the Lord, not perfect, but really doing our best, there is a peace that mutes many uncertainties.

Searching for answers during the darkest of my days, I read Elder Nelson's most recent General Conference words at the time, "Obedience allows God's blessings to flow without constraint. He will bless His obedient children with freedom from bondage and misery."[1] "Bondage and misery" described my condition perfectly, and I desperately wanted to be freed. With a dry erase marker, I wrote Elder Nelson's words on my bathroom mirror, and repeated them several times a day. I said them to myself when it was time for family scripture study, for family prayer, for family home evening, and time for church. None of those things had ever been difficult for me before, but they were when I was suffering from depression. Even though freedom didn't feel possible at the time, I knew the words of the prophets were true and viable.

A list of anything "to do," including covenants, can be overwhelming in the depths of depression. With this in mind, I love and appreciate this anecdote of Elder Bednar's:

> Several years ago I spent a Sunday afternoon with Elder Hales in his home as he was recovering from a serious illness. We discussed our families, our quorum responsibilities, and important experiences.
>
> At one point I asked Elder Hales, "You have been a successful husband, father, athlete, pilot, business executive, and Church leader. What lessons have you learned as you have grown older and been constrained by decreased physical capacity?"

Elder Hales paused for a moment and responded, "When you cannot do what you have always done, then you only do what matters most."

I was struck by the simplicity and comprehensiveness of his answer. My beloved apostolic associate shared with me a lesson of a lifetime—a lesson learned through the crucible of physical suffering and spiritual searching.[2]

The way Elder Brough and Elder Christofferson relate patience to obedience rings true for my experience.

Brothers and sisters, there will be times in our lives when the blessings of guidance seem distant or lacking. For such times of distress, Elder D. Todd Christofferson promised: "Let your covenants be paramount and let your obedience be exact. Then you can ask in faith, nothing wavering, according to your need, and God will answer. He will sustain you as you work and watch. In His own time and way He will stretch forth His hand to you, saying, 'Here am I.'"[3]

I also can't help but think of Samuel's words to Saul: "Hath the Lord as great delight in burnt offerings and sacrifices, as in obeying the voice of the Lord? Behold, to obey is better than sacrifice, and to hearken than the fat of rams" (1 Sam. 15:22).

For me, complete obedience eliminates the variable of my own worthiness from the equation, and gives me the peace that the outcome is in the Lord's hands.

True faith is not based on outcomes, as Shadrach, Meshach, and Abednego so boldly and bravely taught as they faced the burning fiery furnace, "...our God whom we serve is able to deliver us from the burning fiery furnace...*But if not*, be it known unto thee, O king, that we will not serve thy gods, nor worship the golden image which thou hast set up" (Daniel 3:17-18, italics added).

My mother, who was close to me day in and day out for months through all of this said, "Obedience is key and speeds recovery."

By the act of willing your obedience according to your faith, the Lord is bound by His promises (D&C 82:10).

YOU AS THE STEWARDSHIP

CHAPTER 12

❋

"I know our prayers are heard. So, so many people have, and are serving our family...just someone to talk to keeps the darkest thoughts away"

(*My journal*, Sept. 4, 2011).

A loving Heavenly Father knew we would not be at our best all of the time in this test of mortality. Wisely, he appoints stewards in different ways with specific stewardships. A steward is one who attends to the concerns of others. Likely, you are and have been, in many capacities as a steward— some forever, some for a time. For example, as a parent your children are your stewardship; as a ministering brother or sister, those you visit are your stewardship; a Bishop's stewardship are his ward members. Without a stewardship, the steward labors in vain. However, when a "stewardship" accepts love and service, divine lessons are learned, relationships are forged and strengthened, and all are "edified and rejoice together" (D&C 50:22).

President Dieter F. Uchtdorf explained: "Our Father in Heaven knows His children's needs better than anyone else. It is His work and glory to help us at every turn, giving us marvelous temporal and spiritual resources to help us on our path to return to Him."[1]

Those resources absolutely include your Savior, your spouse if you are married, your Bishop, and your ministering brothers and sisters. Those resources may include children and extended family, neighbors, friends, and professionals. Likely, those resources include many on the other side of the veil. Elder M. Joseph Brough speaks of these as "personal care packages" developed to suit each one of us by our loving Heavenly Father. *Receive the care package God has personally assembled for you!* "For what doth it profit a man if a gift is bestowed upon him, and he receive not the gift? Behold, he rejoices not in that which is given unto him, neither rejoices in him who is the giver of the gift" (D&C 88:33).

Elder Brough speaks specifically about the care package found in the priesthood leader called to lead and guide you, your Bishop. He quotes President Packer:

President Boyd K. Packer said: "Bishops are inspired! Each of us has agency to accept or reject counsel from our leaders, but never disregard the counsel of your bishop, whether given over the pulpit or individually."[2]

Searching for answers, I asked my Bishop if I could talk to him. I had served as the Young Women's President under his leadership, and now, sitting across from his large wood desk, I could tell we both felt that *other* vivacious, active, ever-moving young women's leader of just a year or so previous seemed liked a different person. Despite his concern, I could tell he really didn't know what to say. Finally, he asked, "Have you yelled lately?" I think the question took us both a little by surprise. I responded that I had not. I'm not really one that does a lot of yelling. He told me he thought it would be good for me to get it out, that I needed to go somewhere and just yell. Not only was his counsel against my nature, but it seemed like yelling would take a lot of energy I didn't have. However, I had asked for his counsel, and I was resolute in being obedient to it.

Shortly thereafter, my husband drove me out to my parents' house in farm country, a half-hour outside the city. (I didn't want to be yelling in my neighborhood surrounded by neighbors sure to hear and wonder.) I warned my parents about what I was about to do and why, and then I walked down behind the house towards the field. I don't remember what I said, but I yelled it. Honestly, I don't know if this did anything for me other than I knew I was being as obedient as I possibly could to follow the counsel of my Priesthood leader. In a conversation with my Bishop since that time, we have both laughed about that experience. He said that was the strangest counsel he ever gave. Regardless, I knew I had been obedient to the counsel of my priesthood leader, and I knew God knew my effort.

Actually, it is my experience that Bishops are becoming more and more aware of mental health challenges and are better prepared to recommend trusted professional resources if needed. In addition, they preside over the Ward Council where many willing and able people meet to discuss and carry out the service which all members of your family will need. They are inspired as to your welfare. And perhaps above all, Bishops are blessed in a remarkable way to feel God's love for you and can convey that love through words, priesthood keys and blessings.

Ministering brothers and sisters may feel ill-equipped to help with something they may not understand. However, if you communicate and allow them to help with those things that they can do, you will find your burden lifted, and witness, in action, God's perfect order of caring for the one. You also may be surprised to learn that they understand your burden better than you think, or know someone who does. The same applies to friends, neighbors, and others.

I remember clearly the day I called my visiting teacher and told her that the doctor said I could no longer take care of babies at night. Feeling completely broken and inept, in tears I asked her to arrange for someone to help my husband with one of the babies each night. I had never really asked for anything significant from a visiting teacher, and now I was asking for something HUGE. She didn't even hesitate, but asked a few clarifying questions. She made sure someone trusted and loving reported to our home every evening to take care of one of the babies. For 4 months—every night!! Next to this truly selfless act, was that every sister who came to our home acted as though it was a privilege to come cuddle and snuggle with my babies although they were sacrificing their own sleep and comfort, and would be returning home to their own full plate of responsibility the next morning. To this day, I cannot think of these selfless women and their quiet, yet powerful influence on our lives, without great humility and love.

Because there were so many that helped us, and my time was so limited, I resorted to a mass produced thank you card. This is what was written inside:

> Like this card, my life has become very much simplified. I wish I could hand write you these thoughts, but that opportunity may never come.

These words are the words of Sister Julie Beck. When she spoke them, they immediately moved from my ears to my heart and my eyes brimmed with tears. She so perfectly described what I am experiencing in my life right now.

"Every day, Relief Society sisters around the world experience the entire range of mortal challenges and experiences. Women and their families today live face to face with unrealized expectations; mental, physical...illness.... All of these difficulties have the potential to bleach the bones of faith and exhaust the strength of individuals and families.

One of the Lord's purposes in organizing the sisters into a discipleship was to provide relief that would lift them above 'all that hinders the joy and progress of woman.'

I hope my granddaughters will understand that through Relief Society, their discipleship is extended and they can become engaged with others in the kind of impressive and heroic work the Savior has done. The kind of work the sisters of this Church are asked to do in our day has never been too modest in scope or inconsequential to the Lord. Through their faithfulness, they can feel His approval and be blessed with the companionship of His Spirit...I hope my granddaughters will understand that visiting teaching is an expression of their discipleship and a significant way to honor their covenants."[3]

Yours are the hands that have helped to lift my burden and bring the real relief that the Relief Society was meant to provide. I cannot express my gratitude, but I want you to know it runs deep. Yours has been an "impressive and heroic work" in my life. I hope you feel the approval of the Savior and the companionship of His Spirit as that is the greatest of thanks, and what I hope and pray for. The sincerest thank you, Makala

In the ever and ongoing march of time, the tables will be turned, and you as a "steward" will be so much better prepared and armed with empathy and knowledge if you will accept the role of "stewardship" gracefully and humbly now, allowing your stewards to minister to you. There is much to be gained, and you will find your relationships with those who serve much more real and deep.

PART 3

HEALING

"The wound is the place where the Light enters you"

(attributed to Jalaluddin Mevlana Rumi, 13th-century Persian poet).

"...there is no sin or transgression, pain or sorrow, which is outside of the healing power of His Atonement"

(C. Scott Grow, "The Miracle of the Atonement," *Ensign*, April 2011).

"Broken minds can be healed just the way broken bones and broken hearts are healed"

(Jeffrey R. Holland, "Like a Broken Vessel," *Ensign*, Nov. 2013).

PREVENTION IS THE BEST MEDICINE

CHAPTER 13

✷

I cannot find anything in my journal about prevention. I waited too long. Be wiser than I was.

Denying that you have the stomach flu, or feeling you are above that, or you have more control than to let the stomach flu happen to you, rarely, if ever, prevents you from vomiting and spending more time than you would like in the bathroom. Depression is not something that goes away with denial, feeling like you are above being depressed, or that you have more control than to get depressed. It has a physical cause and presence, and can be no more wished away than the stomach flu.

Similar to the stomach flu, accepting it for what it is, and treating it, will decrease the time required to heal. With the stomach flu, if you don't make a conscious effort to keep hydrated, reintroduce mild foods slowly, and get good bacteria into the gut, the discomforts tend to last longer and your normal lifestyle is interrupted longer. Such is the case with depression. The sooner you call it what it is, educate yourself with the help of professionals if necessary, and treat the chemical deficiencies and imbalances, the less time the "discomforts" will last and your normal lifestyle will be interrupted. Unlike the stomach flu which even in worst cases lasts only a couple days, untreated depression can rob you of life's fulfillments and joys for extended periods of time. It can become debilitating and even life- threatening at worst.

In preventing illness whenever possible, watch for the stress indicators in yourself and in others you may be able to help. As with your automobile, be alert to rising temperatures, excessive speed, or a tank low on fuel. When you face "depletion depression," make the requisite adjustments. Fatigue is the common enemy of us all—so slow down, rest up, replenish, and refill. Physicians promise us that if we do not take time to be well, we most assuredly will take time later on to be ill.[1]

So, if life seems a little blah, if you are beginning to notice changes in your eating or your sleeping, if tears come easier than usual, or if you are feeling more and more overwhelmed and exhausted, or on edge, now is the time to give heed to those cues. Take it from me, no one wants to be depressed any more than anyone wants the stomach flu, but doing something about it now will be significantly to your benefit—both personally, and to your family and circle of friends.

KNOWLEDGE
IS POWER

✷

CHAPTER 14

"I have an apt. with Dr. D on Wednesday to

learn about anxiety and this healing process"

(*My journal*, August 22, 2011).

"Diagnosed with postpartum depression

today. Started on medication"

(*My journal*, Sept. 2, 2011).

Despite being the mother of 6 children and having a background as a Registered Nurse, I was extremely deficient in knowledge about depression as a true mental illness, with researched etiologies. Once it was explained to me what was causing the "dark" and the "crazy" I was experiencing—that there are actually chemicals that have names that were depleted, and there are certain things that build those chemicals back up—then I had some power in facing my beast. That's not to say that all of a sudden things changed, and I went gung-ho into the battle. I still looked at my shoes before my daily walk and wondered if I could tie them because of the heaviness I felt. However, knowing there were certain things I could do that would help to heal my mind gave me something to work towards.

For me, googling for information and reading the melting pot of others' experiences on the Internet was NOT a good idea. It didn't take me long to realize that doing my own "research" set my mind reeling and increased my anxiety. I stopped using the Internet. For accurate information pertaining to me, I relied on my health care professionals.

There is another kind of knowledge that is power. That knowledge is the knowledge we have gained from our life experiences and through the Holy Ghost, prior to the crisis we are now experiencing. "We doubt not the Lord nor his goodness. We've proved him in days that are past.'[1] In my journal I wrote:

> I have pondered how important it is for me now to have the knowledge of God and His love because my soul is in such turmoil I often cannot feel it. Mosiah 4:6 & 11 talk about the "knowledge of the goodness of God..." and "knowledge of the glory of God..." How grateful I am for that knowledge (My journal, Sept. 9, 2011).

WHO'S WHO IN MENTAL HEALTH?

CHAPTER 15

✻

"Had an emergency visit with psychiatrist this afternoon. Will start back on [name of medication]. Got referral for endocrinologist"

(*My journal*, Nov. 9, 2011).

The mental health realm of medicine was all new to me. Although I had done a unit on mental health and had been an intern as a student nurse at a juvenile mental health center, entering the stage of mental health as the patient was a whole new ball game. Just figuring out whom to go to for help can be a bit of a puzzle. If it's as new to you as it was to me, here's a quick rundown:

I started with my **family physician** who had been my doctor for 8 years. She was extremely patient with me as I insisted something beyond postpartum depression was wrong with me. A family physician can educate you and prescribe limited medications. A family physician can also refer you to other professionals such as therapists and psychiatrists if you require additional help. Most OB/GYN doctors have training and experience treating post-partum depression as well.

A **therapist** or **counselor** is the one who can sit down with you, learn about your situation and struggles, and teach you cognitive and behavioral skills to help you cope and heal. These visits are often called "sessions," and can occur on an "as needed" basis, usually more often to begin with. They offer a non-judgmental, objective approach.

A **psychiatrist** is a medical specialist for the brain, much like an orthopedic surgeon is a medical specialist for the bones. Unlike the traditional arm of medicine in which data is gathered through laboratory results as well as verbal conversations, most of the data a psychiatrist can gather completely depends upon your conversations with him or her. Thus, it is obviously very important to be completely honest and transparent, as what you say is the entire pool of information from which to work. A psychiatrist's role is largely to figure out the medication(s) that will be of greatest benefit to you. Once again, appointments with psychiatrists will be more often initially, and then less often as you stabilize.

Mental health institutions are facilities reserved for extreme cases in order to protect the individual and others when brain chemicals are so deficient or out of balance that physical well-being is at risk. "Institutions" have quite a negative connotation, but at one point, I was begging my family doctor to admit me, such was the extremity I felt. Mental health institutions play an important role in keeping the whole person safe.

WHAT DO I DO TO GET HEALTHY?

CHAPTER 16

"Talked to Shelly this morning. She assured me I will feel normal again—my body and mind will heal"

(*My journal*, Nov. 7, 2011).

A lot of these ideas may seem like "no-brainers" and we hear them repeatedly in any pursuit of healthy living. Here's why they are important in relation to depression.

Sleep. This topic presents the paradox of depression. That which you need most to restore a healthy brain is what your brain can't seem to do— shut off! The less sleep you get, the more you worry about it, which only makes it more difficult to relax and retreat to that ever-elusive reprieve of dreamland. I was so sleep-deprived because of caring for twins that I didn't recognize any problem with sleep until I just couldn't. My body was so tense I felt as though I was shivering. I was in such a state that my phone call to the doctor resulted in a sleep aid medication. Later, my psychiatrist changed the sleep aid to something he thought would help me to feel more rested and not just knocked out. It worked, and the long haul to recovery finally seemed to be underway. There is some controversy as to the effectiveness of sleep aids. Some people report that sleep medications actually excite their brain instead of relax it. Under the direction of your healthcare provider, you may have to try more than one to have success if a sleep aid is necessary.

Sleep aid medications aren't the only thing that can be done. If you are just beginning to notice symptoms of depression you would wisely look into the "sleep science" that has surged in recent years as Americans complain more and more about difficulty falling asleep and staying asleep. Sleep hygiene refers to a routine and circumstances that surround your sleep. These routines serve to cue your brain that shut-down time is coming soon, and it's time to wind down. Sleep hygiene is different for different people but some common ground includes certain clothes for sleeping, a certain place for sleeping, and a repeated pre-bedtime routine (i.e. washing face, brushing teeth, reading or praying) which occurs at the same time each evening. Most people sleep more soundly in cooler temperatures so adjusting your thermostat may make a difference. Some things that are NOT recommended prior to sleep are big meals, exercising, and electronic use. Some professionals recommend no "blue-light" for

1 ½ hours prior to the time you wish to fall asleep. Reading before bed should be done in low light, but not electronic light. Some people find oils, or chamomile, or melatonin effective; a warm herbal tea before bed is soothing to others.

If you wake during the night, give yourself a certain amount of time to fall back to sleep, but if you start to toss and turn, get up and do something for up to an hour in low light. Keeping things quiet is best. The purpose of this is to distract your mind from the one thing it is wrapped around (not sleeping), but not to excite your mind to the point where it thinks it's time to be in full gear. After a period of being awake but not aroused, try to go back to bed again. I have found that putting something to memory, or working on putting something to memory, as I try to drift off is very helpful. This diverts the mind from the self-destructive, "I can't sleep, I need to sleep. I can't sleep, I really need to sleep!" If nothing else, scriptures and good literature are always a good addition to your mental repertoire.

Getting out of bed each day feels like a millstone around your neck, but don't sleep or lay in bed past a consistent appointed time in the morning, no matter how tired you are or how little sleep you got. If you sleep longer than is needful, your rhythm will be messed up for your attempt the following night. Exercise and physical exertion during the day will contribute to better sleep. God made our bodies and our brains to work.

Eat a balanced diet. The chemicals in our brain that are deficient or "out-of- whack" when we feel the effects of depression are built of protein—amino-acids to be specific. In order for our bodies to replace and rebalance what is lost, they have to have the correct building blocks to do so. Make sure you get enough protein. Protein is found in more places than you think it is, and if you are anything like I was, eating was a chore. If I had a chance of getting anything down it was something "light" or liquid. For example, Greek yogurt has about 17 grams of protein per serving and protein shakes are a good option if you are reduced to liquids. (I lived off of smoothies and protein shakes for what seemed like forever.) "Balanced" diet of course would include fruits and vegetables and plenty of other natural foods. Some research shows that inflammation exacerbates depression. Sugar, refined carbohydrates, and processed foods may increase inflammation in the body, so stay away from those.[1] Eating nutritiously will also prevent other health complications from arising.

Exercise. This is either something you love or hate regardless of struggling with depression. I can't overemphasize the importance exercise is to healing. Exercise plays two major roles. One, as mentioned, our bodies were made to work and when they are worked, they are primed to rest. Exercise increases the chances of good sleep. Two, exercise in and of itself increases the concentrations of the neurotransmitters, brain chemicals, that give us a sense of well-being. The effect is immediate and long-lasting. It feels good to exert whether you are a lover or hater of exercise. Even if you don't consider yourself an exerciser, you can most likely physically walk. Walk. Walk. I'm a jogger, but my weight got down to a point that my doctor told me to just walk. Getting dressed, tying my shoes, and getting out the door was almost more than I could muster the "umph" for, but once I put one foot in front of the other, and then again, it felt liberating. If you are an exercise "hater," solicit someone's help to make you accountable. Maybe this is a walking partner, maybe this is someone who will talk to you on the phone while you walk. It doesn't have to be walking or jogging, there are as many different methods of exercise as there are menu options at the closest restaurant. If anything sounds better than something else, do it. Research shows that anything that makes you sweaty for 20 minutes at least 3 times a week has significant benefits. At bare minimum, stretch and work up from there. After sleeping and eating, exercise is the number one priority.

Simplify. We live in a fast-paced world where unless we are deliberate, family life is overscheduled. Each "to do," each pick-up and drop off, each meeting, each game, each recital, each performance, each engagement of any kind takes planning and energy. What may have been a manageable schedule at one time, is now a peppering of withdrawals on your brain and body. Figure out what is most important and let the other "commitments" go. You will be surprised at what your family will survive without. When you simplify your life, the ledger of your recovery will begin to register more deposits than withdrawals.

Don't isolate yourself. Ann Romney in her book, "In This Together," chronicled her battle with MS, and included in her "afterword" a checklist for dealing with "any bag of rocks." She also recognized this important part of healing and called it, "Make and strengthen connections with others."[2] Making and strengthening connections with others will be one of the last things you feel like doing while struggling with depression.

When I think of this important part of getting well, giving antibiotics to my toddlers comes to mind. None of my kids were even close to cooperative when it came to taking medicine. Burning fevers and aching ears wasn't enough to convince my little ones that the pink liquid in the syringe was the solution to their pain. My husband and I tried ALL tactics from bribery to stealth, but it always came down to one of us physically holding our child down and the other forcing the antibiotic down their throat. It was awful!! But, without fail, they felt better within 24 hours and were almost back to themselves within two days. (When they felt better, it was even harder to get them to finish out the 10 days of pink liquid!!) The reason this comes to mind is because that pink medicine is much like the sociality that exists around us despite what we feel like on the inside. When depression weighs on us, we "kick and scream" to avoid going into public, being around people, and interacting in society. We say to ourselves, "I don't want other people to see me like this." In reality, that pink medicine, that sociality, is going to help you get better. It is going to ease the pain. "...Nearly everyone does better when they avoid isolation and foster social connections" say BYU mental-health experts.[3] I found that to be true. The goal is that the healing process will lead to a flourishing life, and BYU President Kevin J. Worthen has wisely noted, "No one can flourish in isolation."[4]

At first, I had to plan for it. When my sweet aunt called me up to tell me she was coming to pick me up for a pedicure, I couldn't do it. I just couldn't. But, if I agreed to go to dinner with my husband and some friends on a certain day, and wouldn't let myself back out because I knew it was good for me, I would will myself through getting ready and leaving the house. With company that I knew well, getting out was a good thing. I noticed it did two things in particular. First, talking with other people about their lives helped me to forget myself for a little while. That's healthy. Second, acting "normal" leads to being "normal." Like my Missionary Training Center teacher used to remind us over and over again, "Fake it, 'til you make it!"

Use healthy coping mechanisms. Some of the "self-medicating" methods people turn to may bring immediate relief but will do damage in the long run. Obviously, that would include drugs, alcohol, pornography, gambling and the like. Other less obvious methods of negative self-medicating would include video-gaming, binge eating, and excessive sleeping. I emphatically agree with what Elder Ballard said, "Inappropriate technology and social media, including video games...dull your spiritual sensitivity."[5] Evaluate what it is you do to bring relief and ask yourself if it will have long-term positive effects. Here are some ideas for positive coping mechanisms:

‣ *Journal*. This can mean talking through your challenges and frustrations on paper without any threat of being judged. Sometimes the best feedback is no feedback, but just releasing the tension. I remember President Hinckley's daughter, Virginia Pearce coming to the Missionary Training Center to speak to us as missionaries. She talked about the importance of keeping a journal and how doing so helps us to process our lives. I have found that to be true. I kept a daily journal during my dark time. When I finally felt like I had come to the end of the tunnel, I put that journal away. I was honestly afraid of its contents. I didn't open its pages for a few years, not wanting to touch any part of what I had been through. Then I was asked to speak for a group and I got brave and opened its pages. I was astounded; it wasn't dark at all. I wondered how that could possibly be when I knew exactly how I had felt during those days, and weeks, and months. It just goes to show that how we feel when our central nervous system is depressed is not reality.

Just keeping a gratitude journal will do wonders for you. If you have never tried it, simply write down at least one thing a day for which you are grateful. It might be something, someone, or the little miracles along the way. You will be amazed at how keen your eyesight for good becomes.

Previously I noted what BYU Professor Gregory Clark said, "Faith is founded upon our memory of divine witnesses and blessings received in the past and upon our hope in divine promises for the future."[6] Faith can be strengthened as you draw upon past experiences. Read your own journal entries from brighter days. If you didn't record faith-promoting experiences then, write them down now. Additionally, your future faith can be strengthened as you now record the hand of the Lord in your life during a very trying time.

- *Take a walk, outside, in fresh air.* Whether it's hot or cold, or the perfect temperature, there is something invigorating to the soul about a walk in fresh air. My mother-in-law is an accomplished musician and a fan of history's greatest musicians. Searching for a way to help me while two states away, she sent me an iPod shuffle with some of her favorite pieces and I listened to that music on many, many walks. I always felt better walking than wallowing. Even just the boost from the vitamin D from the sun is worth the effort to be outside in the sunshine.

- *Deep-breathing /relaxation techniques/meditation.* I'm not a professional, but not too long ago a friend texted me when she was heading into a panic attack. I simply reminded her to breathe— breathe in deeply until she felt like she could not inhale any more, and then suck just a bit more, and then let it out as slowly as she possibly could. I told her to do it two more times. This does two things—it really does slow a racing heart, and it focuses the mind on making your body do something rather than your body making your mind do something. Your mind may seem like your weakness, but it can also be your greatest strength. Relaxation techniques and meditating are other ways the mind can take control the way you want it to.

‣ *Positive self-talk.* Eliminate the negative expression "I can't" and replace it with "I can". Then act. "I can make the bed." "I can read a story to my child." After my experience, and to keep my nursing license current, I took an online continuing education course on depression. One of the hopeful things I learned from taking that course is that it is quite possible that our behavior can affect our brain chemistry. For example, numerous stressors or traumas may cause a person's brain chemistry to be affected leading to depression, but that same person may learn how to change thoughts and behavior in a way to cope, thus changing brain chemistry and relieving depression.

One major game-changer for me was along these lines of positive thinking. At one point, I realized that instead of being victim to my feelings, I had to take control and make a choice about how I felt. Repeatedly, my eyes would open in the morning and look at the ceiling and a tangible, heavy dread would come over my mind and body as I realized I had to face another day of torture. One morning as this happened yet again, I recognized the trap. It was at that point that I decided to make myself get up at a certain time each morning and get outside for fresh air and exercise first thing. It was a huge change of direction. I made my feelings succumb to my choices instead of letting my choices succumb to my feelings. It was the catalyst that helped to change, "I can't" back into "I can". (It helped to have Lizza waiting for me on the corner a mile away at 5:45 regardless of the weather, all winter long. She hates jogging. Now, that's a friend.)

‣ *Do something creative.* President Uchtdorf has taught, "The desire to create is one of the deepest yearnings of the human soul. No matter our talents, education, background, or abilities, we each have an inherent wish to create something that did not exist before…Creation brings deep satisfaction and fulfillment. We develop ourselves and others when we take unorganized matter into our hands and mold it into something of beauty…"[7]

I can do a little sewing and so Lizza asked me to help her make some decorative pillows for her bed. Before the cloud of depression, I could easily make a pillow in about 15 minutes, start to finish. In the midst of my ordeal, I remember standing at the table over my cutting board with the measurement guide and my rotary cutter for what seemed liked hours. Just cutting out the fabric to the correct dimensions was building the Eiffel tower in my fogged brain, but I kept at it and I did it. I found that doing something creative forced me to focus my mental energy on something outside of myself and gave me periods of time when I was not consumed by the disease.

‣ *Serve.* President Hinckley said, "The best antidote for worry is work. The best medicine for despair is service. The best cure for weariness is to help someone even more tired."[8] If you are a post-partum sufferer of depression you may feel you are in the same trap I felt I was in. I felt as though I couldn't serve anyone because I was tied to two babies who needed me at least every 2—4 hours. There are ways. Pray and be open to ideas. Give away what you create as gifts— double whammy, create and serve. Perhaps getting a babysitter for a few hours so you can go help someone else is the answer.

‣ *Work.* When Adam was being cast out of the Garden of Eden, he was told,"…because thou hast hearkened unto the voice of thy wife, and hast eaten of the tree, of which I commanded thee, saying, Thou shalt not eat of it: cursed is the ground for thy sake; in sorrow shalt thou eat of it all the days of thy life" (Genesis 3:17, italics added). The footnote for "sorrow" references the word "travail." "Travail" is defined as difficult labor or toil. So, as in all God does, He "cursed" the ground so that we can toil in it for our good, for our sake. My sister calls it "dirt therapy." Whatever you call it, the irony of getting dirt under your fingernails is that it produces a cleansing feeling. Whether it's mowing the lawn, raking leaves, weeding the garden, or planting flowers, work is therapeutic. Elder Neal A. Maxwell said, "Work is always a spiritual necessity…"[9] President David O. McKay said, "Let us realize that the privilege to work is a gift, that power to work is a blessing, that love of work is success."[10] Good, hard work will aid your journey back to health and happiness.

‣ *Get Moving, stay moving.* I was reading a children's book to my kids the other night called, *The Rhino Who Swallowed a Storm*. I had just grabbed a handful of books at the library for a little storytime variety, not realizing the book's content. The book is actually about the healing process after tragedy and one couplet reminded me of one of my observations during the crisis period. "It doesn't much matter if you're fast or you're slow, if you want to move forward, just trust and let go."[11] I was reminded that as impossible as it was to sometimes get going, once I got going, the going got easier. I noticed that once I was busy about the tasks of the day, there was a "lightening" that occurred. The heaviness seemed to lift somewhat as I kept moving. Though I'm not a physicist, Sir Isaac Newton's law seems very relevant, "Every object persists in its state of rest…unless it is compelled to change that state by forces impressed on it." That impressing force requires a great deal of compelling yourself, but once put in motion, motion isn't as difficult.

An attempt to implement all of these at once is as good as throwing in the towel when the simple basics of life are overwhelming. The truth is that getting healthy takes effort and work. When Sheri Dew asked Elder Nelson what he learned about his experiences trying to forward the work of the church against insurmountable odds in Eastern Europe, he responded, "that the Lord likes effort."[12] Pick one of these ways to promote your health, take one day at a time. When my dad taught me to ride a bike, he told me not to look at the front wheel but to look at the horizon. It was like magic for my balance. Right now, for your balance, my counsel is to stay focused on the front wheel and only take a peak at the horizon from time to time. One day at a time is plenty to take on. Elder Scott states success indeed comes one day at a time, "We **become** what we want to **be** by consistently **being** what we want to **become** each day."[13] Incremental changes consistently will yield monumental results.

DO I NEED THERAPY?

CHAPTER 17

✳

"Took [therapist's] advice and just kept moving today"

(*My journal*, Oct. 22, 2011).

"Therapy" by definition is "the treatment of disease or disorders, as by some remedial, rehabilitating, or curative process."[1] That definition includes all forms of therapy, including medicinal, but here we will use the term "therapy" as the kind of "curative process" which occurs when you, who are suffering from depression, have open and confidential conversations with someone trained to assist those with mental illnesses. These mental healthcare professionals are called "therapists" and can be significant contributors to your "curative process."

A trained professional therapist offers an objective outlook on your personal situation. The therapist will help you to see and understand things clearly as opposed to the way you feel about things under the cloud of depression. Therapy can give you practical tools on how to reframe negative thinking, offer behavioral skills, and teach coping strategies for anxiety. If there are underlying issues that contribute to depression or exacerbate it, therapy can help you work through those as well. If you have never been a part of professional therapy before, that new encounter may seem large and looming in and of itself. Sue Bergin of the BYU Magazine gives great suggestions about "making therapy work for you." Here are some of them:

- Start with recommendations. Remember you don't have to stay with the first therapist you try.

- A good therapist lets you talk and helps you find your own solutions. If a therapist is doing most of the talking, you may need another therapist.

- You should feel comfortable with the therapist and feel that he or she is not judgmental and not confrontational. You should feel understood.

- A good therapist is invested in your well-being. He or she cares how you're doing and if you're getting better.

- Keep in mind that therapy is not a quick fix. Sometimes

people get worse before they get better.

▸ Choose someone who understands and respects your values. That doesn't mean your therapist must be LDS, but the therapist should encourage you to talk about the spiritual aspects of your life and be willing to learn about your values to better help you.[2]

I think a better name for a therapist is a "coach." We welcome and seek out good coaches in all aspects of our lives. Athletic coaches, financial coaches, even life coaches, as well as tutors, Bishops, accountants, dentists, doctors, and business consultants to name a few. We seek out the counsel of all these different people because they have experience and expertise in a specific subject. *They can see where we are and help us get to where we want to be with their wisdom and our effort.* On the basketball court, a player sees the game from his or her perspective. While that perspective can be valuable, it doesn't compare to the coach's perspective. The coach sees the big picture. The coach is watching all the players in the game, offense and defense. The coach can see what is working and what isn't working. He knows the strengths and weaknesses of each of his players. The coach calls plays and makes adjustments in response to specific circumstances. When players respond to good coaching, progress is made and incredible victories can take place. Good therapists play the role of a good coach in mental health. They see the big picture, all the players, obstacles, strengths and weaknesses. The therapists calls the plays and recommends adjustments in your specific circumstances. When you respond to good coaching, progress is made and incredible victories can take place. *Good therapists can see where you are and help you get to where you want to be with their wisdom and your effort.*

I really appreciate what Randy Pausch, author of *The Last Lecture*, had to say about therapy. After being diagnosed with terminal pancreatic cancer and given 4—6 months to live, he and his wife decided to see a counselor. In Pausch's words, "I had spent much of my life doubting the effectiveness of counseling. Now with my back against the wall, I see how hugely helpful it can be. I wish I could travel through oncology wards telling this to patients who are trying to tough it out on their own."[3]

To answer the question, "Do I need therapy?" consider these thoughts: Therapy can be helpful in and of itself, independent of other interventions. Therapy has also been shown to increase the effectiveness of other interventions such as medicine. Other healthcare professionals may recommend you see a therapist, or you may just feel that an objective point of view may prove beneficial. If you are in need of coping or grounding skills to deal with anxiety or find yourself trapped in a downward spiral of negative thoughts, therapy can provide you with tools to change your habits in the way you think. If one or more of these thoughts ring true for you, a trusted therapist may be your next step on your road of healing.

I would say the same thing Pausch wished he could tell everyone, therapy can be "hugely helpful" and you don't have to try and tough it out on your own.

DO I NEED MEDICATION?

CHAPTER 18

✷

"Today I am grateful for...medication..."

(*My journal*, Oct. 10, 2011).

Before my own experience, my understanding of antidepressant medication was inaccurate. I'm a firm believer in "you choose your own happiness" and the term "anti-depressant" seemed to be a pill making that choice. Actually, anti-depressants are medications that help to bring your brain chemistry back into balance so you can make the choice of your own happiness.

The following comes from WebMd, and summarizes very well what I learned and experienced about anti-depressant medication:

> ...Depression is one of the most treatable mental disorders. Between 80% and 90% of people who have it benefit from treatment. The kind of management you need depends on your specific situation, but for some people, medication can be very helpful.

> That's because brain chemistry may contribute to the condition, so taking antidepressants can actually change your brain chemistry and help you feel better.

> The most common antidepressants are called selective serotonin reuptake inhibitors (SSRIs). They're considered relatively safe and cause fewer side effects than other kinds of medications used to treat depression.

> How Do SSRIs Work?

> SSRIs work by enhancing the function of nerve cells in the brain that regulate emotion. Information is communicated between your brain cells with signals. The chemical messengers that deliver these signals are called neurotransmitters. Serotonin is one type of neurotransmitter.

> When these brain cells (called neurons) send signals to one another, they release a little bit of a neurotransmitter so that the message can

be delivered. They then have to take back the neurotransmitter they released so they can send the next message. This process of replacing the neurotransmitter is called "reuptake."

If you're struggling with depression, the areas of your brain that regulate mood and send messages using serotonin might not function properly. SSRIs help make more serotonin available by blocking the reuptake process. This allows serotonin to build up between neurons so messages can be sent correctly. They're called "selective" serotonin reuptake inhibitors because they specifically target serotonin.[1]

Another class of anti-depressant medication is called SNRIs and this class works not only on the neurotransmitter serotonin, but also on the neurotransmitter, norepinephrine. In some cases, this class of medication is more effective for the person suffering from depression.

Unlike, other medications that can be titrated (measured and adjusted) with blood checks (i.e. blood thinners or thyroid medications), anti-depressants cannot. This fact can make finding the right medication and dosage very tricky. My mood and well-being were so out of whack, "normal" was hard to define. I found myself asking, "Is the way I'm feeling a result of the medication, or the result of something else I'm doing?" The questions seemed like a revolving door never letting me into the room of peace and security. Medication changes are often very rocky roads to travel and oftentimes, symptoms get worse with medication changes before they get better. Such was my case, and after the first medication change, I decided if the medication could get me to a point where I could eat and sleep then I would stick with it and work with it until I was well again.

Another important thing to know about anti-depressants is that they act much differently than other medications, such an antibiotic. Consider the contrast. When you have a bacterial infection and you take an antibiotic, you do so at specific times first to initiate the bacteria-killing substance into your blood stream, and then to keep it at a certain level to maintain the battle against the bacteria. Once the infection is gone, you no longer need the antibiotic and you simply stop taking it. Within a short amount of time, the medication is no longer in your system. Anti-depressants work much differently. It takes a significantly longer period of time for the medication to take effect, even longer for it to reach its peak effectiveness—usually 4-6 weeks for full effect. Depending on the seriousness of your depression, this can seem like an eternity. (Another reason to be aware and not delay help if you suspect you may be suffering from depression.) Anti-depressant medication can also cause an increase in suicidal thoughts prior to effectiveness—this must be noted and prepared for. Anti-depressants cannot be stopped immediately. Your healthcare professional will help you to wean your dosage at a safe rate if you no longer require medication. If you suffer from long-term depression or another mental illness, God be thanked for the day and age in which we live that man has been inspired to create a substance that can bless your life in remarkable ways.

I was also very worried about the idea that I could become dependent or addicted to these medications that had been prescribed. When I expressed my concern, the doctor told me, "if you don't want to be addicted to them, you won't be, they aren't habit-forming." Although I still had my doubts, his statement proved true. There were no cravings or desperate need for more meds. When it was time to discontinue or wean medications, I had no problems. It has also been shown that other therapies in conjunction with medication can increase effectiveness.

For a girl who looked down upon "happy pills," I can honestly say there is a good chance I may not be here today without the benefits of medication.

So to answer the question, "Do I need medication?" The most sound counsel is found in the *For the Strength of Youth* pamphlet:

Your emotional health is...important and may affect your spiritual and physical well-being. Disappointment and occasional sadness are part of this mortal life. However, if you have prolonged feeling of sadness, hopelessness, anxiety, or depression, talk with your parents and your bishop and seek help. In all aspects of your life, seek healthy solutions to problems. Do all you can to safeguard your physical and mental health so you can fulfill your divine potential as a son or daughter of God.[2]

As previously mentioned, I would caution against googling your own diagnosis and therapies. I've found through my own experience, and the experiences of others, that this usually leads to more confusion and anxiety than answers. Work with a trusted professional, and press forward.

HEALING

TAKES

TIME

CHAPTER 19

"Dr. D said it's just a long road but I'm

headed in the right direction"

(*My journal*, Oct. 17, 2011).

"Counselor told me recovery will be like

recovering from pneumonia—slow but steady.

4 to 10 months. Definitely hoping for four"

(*My journal*, Oct. 20, 2011).

Four weeks to the day after our third baby, I had surgery to remove pregnancy-related tumors. I was left with a 5-inch scar that was raised off my skin like a thick bead of caulk. It was rock hard and because of the extent of tissue removal, the area around it was a bit deformed and numb—no sensation. When the wound healed, I thought that scar would be the mark I was left with. Over the course of months and years, that scar has slowly softened and faded, and the feeling has returned to the surrounding area. I have been amazed watching and feeling this very slow process. Not only do I marvel at this body, the greatest of God's creations, but I am deeply grateful for the continued healing He has programmed into our bodies.

In eternity, time itself will be something very different from what we know now: life against the clock. Time in mortality is a very real and active dimension of our lives. Interestingly, time passes different in relation to how we feel. "Time flies when you're having fun" is a real thing when we have been having such a good time we look at the clock and can't believe how much time has passed. On the other hand, when we are beyond bored in a classroom, we all know the feeling of staring at the clock, wondering if it can possibly tick the seconds away any slower. Under the cloak of depression, even the classroom clock ticks fairly quickly in comparison. Depression's time seems like a dimension all of its own—minutes seem like hours, hours like days, and days like years.

The healing process slowly reverses that phenomenon...slowly. The "really bad days" become less and less frequent. The clock ticks a little faster. My family doctor told me early on that in her experience, it usually took about the same time to get out of it, as it did to get into it, including the pregnancy. That information wasn't very welcome at the time, but it proved to be pretty accurate.

The deep healing takes time as well. Our minds automatically associate places and things with our feelings experienced in those places, and with those things. Our brain does this as a defensive mechanism in order to help us avoid repeated, future pain. My agony was postpartum, and so my brain associated its pain with babies. As a result, when I learned anew of a family expecting a baby, I literally felt sick to my stomach. When I held my newborn niece for the first time in November, I had this feeling that she was a bomb just about to explode and ruin her family's life. I knew these were inaccurate and illogical feelings, but they were real feelings just the same. For you, it may not be babies, it may be a specific place, a certain person, or even a repeated time of day, or year, or season. Recognizing these associations and learning to re-think is part of the healing process.

These associations can be very powerful and difficult to change. Therapy is one of the tools that can help in learning to disassociate illogical patterns of thinking.

I believe another vital component is simply time. Time can be our enemy, and yet the constant, never-ceasing passage of time seems to play a significant healing role. This of course is dependent upon the cessation of the stressor. (i.e. Healing from abuse can't take place until the abuse has ceased.) Healing also is contingent upon us doing our part pressing forward.

With the right tools and time, the negative associations I experienced became less and less intense. I can again joy in the announcement of a new baby, and I can again nuzzle in baby cheek chub, and savor the smell of a newborn baby.

There were also things I thought would be forever lost because they were supposed to happen in the window of life when I was just "not happening." Some of those things I felt extremely guilty about. One such example involved our 5-year-old daughter. She was a kindergartener and although she was well prepared for school, I didn't have the time or focus to spend with her reading like I did my older two boys when they were in kindergarten. In addition to my own struggles with depression, the chaos of having 6 kids age 10 and under just made for sheer "survival mode" around our house. Previously, with my older boys, the time we sat and read together was cherished one-on-one time, and the experience itself was as valuable as what reading together did for them educationally. They both soared as readers and LOVED it. It wasn't the same for my sweet girl. Because of the circumstances, reading together was never cherished one-on-one time, IF it happened at all. She didn't learn to read as quickly, and what really hurt my heart, is that she fought it. I felt I had done her a great disservice, one that would continue to penalize her as she grew. One thing I started praying for early on was healing, healing for me and for my family. I have come to know and witness that answered prayer. "... Unto you that fear my name, shall the Son of Righteousness arise with **healing in his wings**; and ye shall go forth and grow up..." (Malachi 4:2, 3 Nephi 25:2). That prayer continued for months and years. As I healed, I was able to have more time and energy (although incrementally) to help our daughter read. She still didn't like it, for years, but we kept at it. It has only been within the last year that she has begun to read because she wants to read. Just last night, she was dancing around elated that it had only taken 4 days to read a lengthy book. A child learning to read may be a poor general example because some kids (and adults) never enjoy reading, and I understand that. However, for me, my daughter's attitude towards reading, and her ability to read is a sure witness of healing.

FROM

MY

SPOUSE

CHAPTER 20

✳

"I love you more than I can possibly show.

I'm so grateful for you. I am here for you→

*for time **and** all eternity. I expect to take full*

advantage of both of those. Love, James"

(a note James left in my journal, Sept. 4, 2011).

"James is the hand of the Lord in my life.

He is continually positive and upbeat"

(*My journal*, Dec. 5, 2011)

Although I'm writing this from the perspective of a husband of one who suffers from depression, the principles in this chapter would also apply to a wife of a husband who suffers, or a parent or friend of someone suffering.

Watching your spouse slip into the dark depths of despair, anxiety, and depression can have its own toll on you. Although you love your spouse and may have served and stood by her side for years or decades, you may feel helpless, confused, and unsure what to do. I know, I've been there.

At times, in an effort to protect you, or maybe even to keep you from thinking less of her, your spouse may not share the deepest and most scary parts of her suffering with you. She may even feel that she is a burden to you and that perhaps you won't want her. Reassure her in word and deed that you love her, are still by her side, and that you aren't going anywhere. When you were married, you committed yourself to your spouse for eternity.

I'm sure some of the darkest moments my wife didn't share with me, but she knew that I would always listen and that she could trust me for help and comfort. I believe she shared most things with me, but even those she didn't share I knew she would if she felt she needed to. I tried not to disregard, play off, or minimize her comments or concerns. I wanted her to keep talking to me. Some thoughts are not rational, but seem logical to a person suffering with depression. You can be the balance, and the calm and patient reassuring voice. If your spouse hints or suggests that they are a burden or apologizes, you can be the reassuring voice that you love her and are glad to be with her.

Encourage your wife to get help. Your sincere desire is for her health, safety, and happiness. Express that you aren't worried about what anybody else thinks, and she doesn't need to be worried either. She is the heart of the home and family and center of your life and God wants her to be healthy to fulfill that role. He will help to find the way and it most likely will involve the help of other people.

Although she didn't express it at the time, Makala has since told me how grateful she was that I expressed daily that I loved her. She needed to hear these words and know she was valued. She needed words of affirmation—"I'm here, we're going to work through this, I love you." Your wife, like mine, may feel like she has nothing to offer the children—you, like me, can have the opportunity to do some of those things that are so important to her and that she wishes she could do. I got to stay home with my family in the mornings to help get breakfast, fix lunches and drive the older kids to school. I have great memories of driving my two oldest boys to school and the three of us singing Christmas songs at the top of our lungs (it wasn't Christmas time yet) and then realizing the windows were down and the crossing guard was giving us strange looks. I had the privilege of printing pictures of my five-year-old daughter and two-year-old son and making them into paper dolls with various sets of clothes. They felt special! I got to read stories to my children and take naps with them or play in the yard. Some of the greatest memories of my life come from this time which was the most trying time of my life. Take time to record these feelings and little experiences in a journal. They will bless your life and your spouse's life.

I know the reality of the Savior's promise in Matthew 11:28-30 "Come unto me, all ye that labour and are heavy laden, and I will give you rest. Take my yoke upon you, and learn of me; for I am meek and lowly in heart: and ye shall find rest unto your souls. For my yoke is easy, and my burden is light." Coming to Christ and relying on Him is the only way. With Him it is possible, and His burden is light. Life is hard, the gospel is easy. His way improves life and you need to trust Him and endure with Him.

You may feel that you can't take time off work to care for your wife and family. I know this is a hard decision for many reasons. You may need to talk to your Human Resource (HR) department if you have one. There may be options available to help you. One option is the Family Medical Leave Act which allows you to take sick days or personal vacation days to care for your spouse or family member for extended periods of time without endangering your job. This act doesn't give you more time off, but it allows you to use continuous periods of your existing sick days or vacation days without being fired. It may require a doctor's note and some paperwork so remember to talk with your HR department. It was a blessing to me and my family and I hope you will be able to find a solution that can help your family as well.

Although not comparable to the one who is actually suffering, your experience will not be easy either. Perhaps you will feel like I did at some point in time. I had a wonderful wife who was (and is) the love of my life, a happy and precious family I loved to spend time with, a profession I loved and in which I felt fulfillment (teaching released-time seminary), I was working on a masters' degree at the university, and had recently been called to a stake calling and was excited to serve. It was a lot to juggle, but I did pretty well, most of the time. Then in a relatively short period of time we entered crisis mode. My wife was suffering extremely both mentally and physically and almost died several times. My children were handed off to various family members for help. I had to take time off of work and eventually applied for Family Medical Leave. My university studies became more stressed. I was also released from my stake calling after having served less than three months. Additionally, I had to have help from women in the ward who would come into my home and care for one twin while I cared for the other twin during the night. I remembered the story of Job in The Old Testament and how quite rapidly the things that were most precious and valued were taken away from him and he was left in a state most would consider awful. I must admit that I analyzed the situation and wondered what was next for me. I felt I had everything precious, meaningful, and important taken from me, except my testimony and my relationship with the Lord. I worried for my wife. I felt guilty for not being at work, teaching my students and helping them. I was nervous over what was happening at work and felt guilty for shifting the burden to someone else. My family was scattered and I felt I wasn't helping them find happiness as I should. I couldn't care for my own family. My university studies, which represented a significant financial investment, had to take a back seat to other priorities. To top it all off, I was released by the stake president from a church calling where I felt the Lord had trusted me to do His work after only 3 months of service.

One day during our family's struggles, I was reading the Old Testament about Moses and the children of Israel being chased by Pharaoh's army to the banks of the Red Sea. I felt I could relate—I couldn't go back or to either side. In front of me lay an insurmountable barrier and behind me, and rapidly pressing upon me and my family, was sure destruction. I needed a miracle! I needed the waters to part in front of me. I prayed for this and sought for revelation to know how to act and how to advance. I noticed in Exodus 14:20 that God sent a "cloud and darkness to [the Egyptians], but it gave light by night to these [the Israelites]." In addition I noticed that in Exodus 14:21, "the LORD caused the sea to go back by a strong east wind all that night, and made the sea dry land, and the waters were divided." I had never noticed that this great miracle wasn't immediate and took all night. I also noticed the method of the miracle—the wind. I don't like wind. I never have liked wind. It is scary, distressing, threatening, and often ruins my plans. However, in this instance, the wind was used by the LORD to make a path forward. In Exodus 14:13-15 the LORD said, "... Fear ye not, stand still, and see the salvation of the Lord," and "The LORD shall fight for you, and ye shall hold your peace. ...Go forward." I assure you that your prayers are being heard. The LORD does love you and your family and knows you and your situation. He is moving already to your deliverance, but miracles sometimes take long dark nights, clouds, lights in the heavens, and wind. It will come, so trust Him and "Go forward."

F R O M

M Y

F R I E N D

CHAPTER 21

✷

"Lizza has been here almost all day..."

(My journal, September 5, 2011).

"Lizza here all day"

(My journal, September 8, 2011).

"For my exercise I walked to Lizza's

house for my daily 'therapy'"

(*My journal*, September 13, 2011).

"Lizza brought balloons for Sariah's birthday"

(*My journal*, October 10, 2011).

"Lizza went with me to James's

seminary class 'to get out'"

(*My journal*, Oct. 20, 2011).

"Lizza helped me take Rex and Lyle

for 6 month check-up..."

(*My journal*, Nov. 20, 2011).

Me: Lizza will never toot her own horn when it comes to the quiet ways she constantly watches out and cares for people. Although there were scores of women who made significant sacrifices to serve our family, Lizza saw it all from start to finish. Whenever she was with me there was a sense of security and I never felt judged. One day as she walked away from our front door down the sidewalk to leave, I distinctly remember thinking that I would not be surprised if she were to dissipate into thin air so angelic was her service. Writing this chapter was difficult for her not only because writing isn't her favorite thing to do, but because she simply doesn't boast about her ways of serving. She agreed to it at my request that there are many out there who want to help, but don't know how. Here are a few excerpts from my journal that give a glimpse of how Lizza was present wherever I needed help. Often, she knew what I needed better than I did. I call it her "sixth sense."

Lizza: My first memory of Makala was at church. She had four cute children all dressed nice. She was always well put together and seemed to have everything under control. I worked with her in Young Womens and was always amazed at how clean her house was. Her children were always well behaved. I admired her knowledge of the gospel and the drive to serve others. As we served alongside each other in this calling we became closer and it turned into a friendship. I loved being around her even though I felt intimated by her and how well she was doing the mom/wife stuff. Our families would get together for BBQs and just to hang out.

Me: I will interject here. For the three months of summer between the time the twins were born and the time I crashed, our poor kids were homebound because we simply couldn't go anywhere. Some of the time they spent with Grandpa and my youngest sister out on the farm, but when they were home, several times a week, Lizza would show up at the door or text and say, "We're headed to the park, would your kids like to come?" "We're headed swimming, I'll come get the kids." "I am on my way to get the kids, we are headed to the movies." Lizza gave my kids a summer that year! I don't know how she did it, but she toted 8 kids under the age of 10 all over that summer, 7 of which are boys! What she may not have realized is she endeared each of my children to her forever!!

Lizza: In August, I got a call from Makala while my family and I were visiting family in Utah. Makala rarely called, we would text but not call. So, I knew something was up. As I listened to what was happening my first thought was, "oh no, I'm not there! How am I going to help her?" She was crying and I could feel she was desperate for some help. Before this, she and James had the twin baby routine under control. Even though it was extremely difficult they were handling it and didn't seem to want help. It had all changed that weekend. I called a friend that we both knew and had twins a couple years earlier. She went over and spent the day with Makala, talking to her and holding babies. It was such a relief that I could call on someone to help when I couldn't be there. I even contemplated flying home early or driving home early to be there, but we waited until we were scheduled to leave Utah. As soon as we got back I raced over there so desperate to see her face and how it was going. I could see just by looking at her she was scared and needed help.

I went over to her house as much as I could, I had 4 little boys at the time so I would wait for my husband to get home or ask a friend to watch my boys. Most days I was there I was holding a baby. But when they were both sleeping I didn't want to just sit around. Makala had told me later on that it was a comfort just to have me there. I would look around to see what would be helpful. I would read books to the older children that weren't in school, fold laundry, do the dishes and most often would sit with Makala in the sun. It was so hard to see someone you grew to love struggle just to eat an apple.

Going over there wasn't always easy. Most of the time I felt uncomfortable especially in the beginning. Isn't that what service is? Going outside your comfort zone to help those in need. My comfort was making dinner for people. That was always easy for me. But that is not what this family needed. I had to observe and ask what would be helpful, but most of the time I just showed up and did it.

Feeling needed was a good feeling but I knew I was needed at home. It was a hard, careful balance. I had to talk to my husband, Zach, after I realized that I was going to be there more, that I wanted to be there. I told him what was going on and that I needed his love and support for me to help my friend. At first it was hard for him and he didn't understand why I was there so much. As time went on he recognized the blessings our family was receiving with me being over there so much and how much I was helping this family and it softened his heart. Makala and James were always showing their gratitude to Zach. They were very aware of the fact that I could not have been there as much if it wasn't for Zach being at home with my boys.

When Makala was getting better I wasn't there as long or as often but I would stop by frequently because you can't tell how someone is doing unless you are looking at them. Makala was comfortable enough to say sometimes, "I would really love for you to stay." Sometimes I would have to change my plans and I wouldn't make it the gym or something, but isn't that what service is? Sacrifice? Someone who used to be so independent and didn't seem to need any help arriving at a place where she would ask for it was a huge change and a change for the better that blessed both of our lives.

Here's one funny little story. Before Makala "crashed" as we call it, I watched the babies one night while James took the kids to a baseball game and Makala was trying to catch some sleep. I told Makala I would wake her up when the babies needed her. James and the kids got home from the game and James tried to get me to leave but I just told him, "no, I will come and get you when they wake up." When they finally woke up at 3am, I left for home. (*Me:* They NEVER slept that long! Lizza is known as "the baby whisperer.") On my way home, no one was on the streets so I didn't make a complete stop at a stop sign and a cop pulled me over. He said, "you know I had to pull you over right?" I replied, "Yeah, sorry I know I didn't stop all the way but I was at a friend's helping with twin babies." He let me go without even asking for my registration.

Me: Lizza never reacted in a way that made me feel like a burden. Although I didn't want to take advantage of her generosity, because of her willingness to help, I knew to whom I could turn when I just couldn't handle life on my own. One year later, to the week, my husband was away to his annual training meeting. The twins got sick with fevers and I didn't sleep much for a couple nights. I laid down one afternoon to try and catch a short nap and even though I was exhausted, I couldn't sleep. The anniversary of my "crash" and not being able to sleep triggered anxieties I hadn't dealt with for months. Who came to the rescue? Lizza. She took one of the twins for a night, and my mom took the other and I got a good night's sleep to break the cycle.

The bond that we developed because of Lizza's selflessness if beyond the category of friendship. We still laugh and cry over those days, and we treasure what we both became because of them.

There are ways to be a true minister, to be the Savior's hands, to those suffering from depression. Be willing to be uncomfortable. Be willing to be present at the sacrifice of self. Be willing to do the uncommon. You will find you are uncommonly blessed for doing so.

THEREFORE, WHAT?

CHAPTER 22

✵

"Really got myself worked up this morning. Couldn't
get my mind off the fact I won't be myself again.
Lizza talked to me about letting the 'old Makala'
go. I think I needed to hear that. I think that's what
makes me anxious and spiral [into crazy thoughts]"

(*My journal*, October 7, 2011).

"One of the ladies I've talked to who has been through something similar said, 'when the good days come, life will have never felt so sweet'"

(*My journal*, Oct. 19, 2011).

"Now no chastening for the present seemeth to be joyous, but grievous: nevertheless afterward it yieldeth the peaceable fruit of righteousness unto them which are exercised thereby" (Hebrews 12:10).

I've heard it said that near the conclusion of council meetings, President Packer would ask those present, "Therefore, what?" To me, this question simply, but powerfully, probes, "after all, what difference does it make?" For President Packer, his intent was to prompt the meeting's members to action—after all we've discussed, what are we going to do about it? I believe we would do well to ask ourselves this question. What am I going to do with the tutoring God has given me through test and trial?

Often quoted, but ever powerful is Elder Orson F. Whitney's observation about trial and suffering. It bears repeating here.

> No pain that we suffer, no trial that we experience is wasted. It ministers to our education, to the development of such qualities as patience, faith, fortitude and humility. All that we suffer and all that we endure, especially when we endure it patiently, builds up our characters, purifies our hearts, expands our souls, and makes us more tender and charitable, more worthy to be called the children of God ... and it is through sorrow and suffering, toil and tribulation, that we gain the education that we come here to acquire.[1]

Therefore, what?

As a result of what you are experiencing or what you have experienced, what eternal education have you gained? What spiritual qualities have you developed? What do you feel now that is exclusive to this challenge that will bless the lives of those around you?

My list is long, some of it can be put into words and some cannot. At the top of the list is the same "therefore, what" that Nephi gained from his hardships, "I know in whom I have trusted. My God hath been my support" (2 Nephi 4:20). Isn't it interesting that different people can learn the same lessons in very different ways? Such a phenomenon is another testament to God's infinite wisdom in helping us to become who He knows we can be. God knows that if we can come to fully trust Him, regardless of our mortal ups and downs, he can mold us into our greatest self.

I'll name a few of the "therefore-what"s from my experience.

I am so much less judgmental. People saw me at my worst. My very worst emotionally. My very worst physically. I looked horrible. I felt horrible. My inclination was to hide from the world, but as circumstances were, my door was revolving—there were people coming and going constantly. I had no choice but to let go of whatever qualms I had about whatever anybody thought about me. Letting that go simultaneously removed my judgment of others. And you know what? They kept coming; they kept loving; they kept lifting. I can easily give people the benefit of the doubt after having walked through the valley of depression.

I became more real. I gained a knowledge in a very profound way that everybody, at one time or another, really struggles. Really, really struggles, and deals with tough stuff. Sometimes struggles may be apparent visually, but more often than not, struggles are hidden. When people really struggle, really hurt, I feel like I know what they feel—at least to a greater degree than before. Somehow, my experience caused me to drop pretenses in reaching out to people. Elder Pingree describes this well, "Like the Savior, whose atoning sacrifice enables Him to succor us, we can use knowledge gained from difficult experiences to lift, strengthen, and bless others."[2] Elder Pingree also notes that Paul obviously spoke from experience as well, "[God] comforteth us in all our tribulation, that we may be able to comfort them which are in any trouble, by the comfort wherewith we ourselves are comforted of God" (2 Corinthians 1:4).

I also became more real in the sense that I am more comfortable being less than perfect. People loved me and reached out to me when I was a mess!! I don't have to be perfect, or pretend to be perfect, or anything like unto. I can accept others the way they are and expect others will do the same to me. And when they don't, that's okay too.

Relationships and friendships strengthened. Jeffery R. Holland quotes James Thurber as saying *"Love is what you go through together."*[3] I believe that was marital advice, but it applies to all relationships. Anybody who has experienced something significant with someone can attest to that truth. For example, if you have ever been on a vacation with someone you share experiences together on that vacation that belong solely to you, and as a result you develop a connection. When you experience something with someone, a certain bond is developed. The more significant the experience, the deeper the bond. How do you think those destitute saints who were carried across the frozen Sweetwater River felt about the Valley boys? I came away from my experience with depression with bonds forged in my own rescue.

Sweet became sweeter. Having tasted bitter, all the little niceties of life are that much more welcome and savored: sunrises and stars, laughter and singing, hugs and handshakes. I suppose it is the law of opposition. Alma said it best, "there could be nothing so exquisite and so bitter as were my pains. Yea, and again I say unto you...that on the other hand, there can be nothing so exquisite and sweet as was my joy" (Alma 36:21).

Focus. Like Elder Hales told Elder Bednar, when you can't do what you've always done, you just do what's important. My depression caused our family to shave life down to what was really important. Since then, I've worried less about what isn't important. I can more clearly see what really matters and where and in what to put my energy. President Monson has said, "I believe that among the greatest lessons we are to learn in this short sojourn upon the earth are lessons that help us distinguish between what is important and what is not."[4]

I've realized what an intense crucible of learning that time was for me. I've continued to learn from that experience with passing time as I have pondered, processed, and studied. As I read the scriptures, think about the words to the hymns, listen to the messages of prophets and apostles, and listen to those around me, "I get it" more than I ever have before. Don't let this education be in vain for you. Be conscientious and intentional about what the Lord has taught you, and what you have learned, and what you are going to do about it. You may never be the same again. And that may be a very good thing.

C O N C L U S I O N

CHAPTER 23

✸

Dave Ramsey is one of my favorite people to listen to on the radio. If you have never heard one of his financial talk shows, broadcasting from Nashville, Dave has an air of southern hospitality and a Tennessee accent. One of the things I love about his show is that he is straightforward and to the point. Even though he doesn't beat around the bush, he is respectful and pleasant to listen to. He also shamelessly speaks of his Christian values as a part of his life and of his profession.

One of the things Dave repeatedly says is, "If you keep doing what you are doing, you will keep getting what you are getting." He generally applies this idea to his callers in the way they are handling their money. If they don't change something about the way they handle their money, they will keep getting the same results, they will be broke and in debt. I have thought about his words often and believe they apply to all walks of life. If you keep doing something over and over again you'll keep getting the same result (scientists actually like that, they call it "proof"). If I keep going to bed too late, I will keep fighting the "snoozies" during the day.

When we want something in our lives to change, we have to do something differently, or the result just keeps repeating itself.

Whether you are beginning to notice the first signs of depression, or whether you have been fighting a long-fought battle, the key to a different outcome is to change something. Change is rarely if ever easy, so what really is the clincher here, is how badly you want a different result. Is the desire for change powerful enough to outweigh the inconvenience, the embarrassment, the pride or whatever else is stopping you? How badly do you want something different from what you have already experienced, or different from what I have described in this book? Change may mean opening up to your spouse or friend about what you are experiencing. Change may mean going through the work of finding a therapist who really helps you. Change may mean actually doing something different about your sleep, your diet, or your exercise. Change may mean having an open conversation with your healthcare professional about what you are feeling and what medications there are to help. Whatever route you feel is your next step, it is the first step to a different outcome. Like I said before, "hard" is redefined by depression, and God can make up the difference between your capabilities and what it takes to get better, if you do your part and let Him in. He wants you well, to be able to feel his light and love in your life... abundantly!

Alma the Younger described coming to Christ in a very profound and intense way through his experience with repentance. I feel my experience, although not deep repentance, brought me to Christ in a very profound and intense way. I echo his words, "My soul hath been redeemed from the gall of bitterness... I was in the darkest abyss; but now I behold the marvelous light of God. My soul was racked with eternal torment; but I am snatched, and my soul is pained no more" (Mosiah 27:29).

E P I L O G U E

I was really hoping there would NEVER be an epilogue to my story.

By the end of the summer of 2018 the manuscript for this book was done, it had been read and edited by several supporters, I had obtained intellectual permissions for the works cited, photos had been taken for the cover, and I had begun working with Josh who would bring it all together as the graphic designer. I felt like I had been guided to bring light from my darkness in the hopes of helping others. That summer life was so good that I remember kneeling by my husband for prayers one night and voicing to him, "Life is so good, when it's over I'm going to miss it."

All of that came to a grinding halt in September when one night turned into my worst nightmare—a repeat of my crash. After a priesthood blessing at 2:30am and about 2 ½ hours of sleep, I woke the next day entirely and completely overwhelmed with the exact mental, emotional, and physical feelings I had experienced 7 years previous. The heaviness, the repulsion to food… all of it. What happened? There were no new babies, I was not sleep deprived, what happened? I was NOT doing this again and I dug in my mental, emotional, and spiritual heals. NO! NO! NO! I had been doing ALL the things that I had learned to fight depression and anxiety—there was no reason for this. I was determined this would be short lived, very short lived because of all that I had learned and thought I knew. But I began to search and dig once again. Why did this happen? My consuming question though was, "God, where did you go overnight?"

The journey could be a whole additional book, twice maybe three times as extensive. Suffice it to say that I searched far and wide. I read books about hormones, diets, the brain, therapies, and others' experiences. I visited doctors of all kinds of medicine, some in distant cities. I went to therapists of all sorts. Chiropractors, natural healers, specialists. I was on a first name basis with the phlebotomist. I had ultrasounds on my abdomen, 24 hour urine tests for heavy metals, injections to test my adrenal glands... I tried several different medications and a whole slew of vitamins and supplements. Nothing changed, at least not for the better. I prayed and pleaded. I searched the scriptures, the Ensign, conference talks, and devotional messages. I had priesthood blessings, I went to church, I fulfilled my calling, and increased my temple attendance. I even spoke in church when I felt I had no testimony to bear. I was pretty sure my name was on the prayer roll continually by those who cared. It seemed as though my list of questions grew ever longer and my list of answers never changed... always nothing. Nothing changed. Every day was the same. I felt sick, anxious, tired. Every day was a battle to get enough calories down (and stay down) to survive. There I was again, in my mind's eye, hanging off the cliff, my fingers digging into a slipping surface all the while going through the motions of being a wife and mother, trying to be "normal." One by one, all the health care professionals in essence threw up their hands and said, "I don't know what the problem is and I don't know how to help you."

What happened to "ask and ye shall receive, knock and it shall be opened unto you?"

Doubts and fears surfaced. Fears about doubts occupied my thoughts. Was it true? Was it real? What is real? What is true? I knew what I had believed all my life. Why did it seem that all my former life experience was up in the air? My life centered on the gospel of Jesus Christ had been happy and rewarding. I hadn't changed anything I was doing, why had the way I was experiencing life changed so dramatically?

In my search, two statements seemed to settle in my soul for pondering, over and over again.

The first was a statement of Wendy Watson's (now Wendy Nelson), in a 1998 BYU Devotional address about change. (I was searching for a big change in my life!) She said, "Through my research with families, I have come to believe that therapeutic change occurs as the belief that is at the heart of the matter is identified, challenged, or solidified (see Lorraine M. Wright, Wendy L. Watson, and Janice M. Bell, Beliefs: The Heart of Healing in Families and Illness [New York: Basic Books, 1996]). [1]

That statement in concert with that of Elder Corbridge's began the change for me, "The challenge is not so much closing the gap between our actions and our beliefs; rather, the challenge is closing the gap between our beliefs and the truth. That is the challenge."[2]

If these statements were true, and I felt that they were, I needed to identify what I believed and close the gap between my belief and the truth to find peace. *So what did I believe that was not true?* Wasn't I searching hard enough? Hadn't I paid the price in effort to get answers?

Exactly 13 months after that first nightmarish night, I woke at 4am, then dozed and dreamed. In that dream I was with my Mom on a trip. We were on our way home and I was packing my things into my carry-on bag. I tucked my boarding pass in my carry-on and continued to gather my things. "It seemed like the more I organized and packed, the more stuff there was. It was time to board and I wasn't done so I sent my Mom on ahead. Even though I didn't feel like my packing was complete, it was time to go so I started looking for my boarding pass where I thought I had put it in my bag. I looked and looked and couldn't find it. Anywhere! I looked through the pages of books, everywhere, several times and couldn't find it. I ended up dumping the contents of my bag and searching and searching. *It seemed the more thorough my search, the more there was to search through.*"[3] There were piles of papers and books, and things to search through, way more than would fit into the carry-on bag. When I woke, the details of the dream remained and so I went to my journal to write. I wanted to know what it meant.

As I've thought about that dream, I understand it at least to some degree. Mom has been on this journey with me the entire way, just like 7 years ago. Over the course of more than a year, she traveled to doctors' appointments by the hundreds of miles. Also, the one, true desire of my heart was to "return home," return to my husband (my true security) and my children, and being the wife and mother I want to be. I was searching for how to get "there," back to my joyful life, in places I would never find it. There were no answers from doctors, therapists, or lab tests. The more I searched the more frustrated I became. There had to be something wrong. And then I realized something. *I believed something was wrong. I believed I had to find out what was wrong and fix it.*

Maybe there was nothing "wrong," maybe this was all "right." Could that be true?

My knee-jerk reaction is "NO! This is NOT right. I feel horrible, physically, emotionally, and spiritually, all day, every day. This is not right."

And then I remembered something a Willie and Martin Handcart Company survivor, Francis Webster, had said,

> "We suffered beyond anything you can imagine and many died of exposure and starvation, but did you ever hear a survivor of that company utter a word of criticism? Not one of that company ever apostatized or left the Church, because everyone of us came through with the absolute knowledge that God lives for we became acquainted with him in our extremities. I have pulled my handcart when I was so weak and weary from illness and lack of food that I could hardly put one foot ahead of the other. I have looked ahead and seen a patch of sand or a hill slope and I have said, I can go only that far and there I

must give up, for I cannot pull the load through it. I have gone on to that sand and when I reached it, the cart began pushing me. I have looked back many times to see who was pushing my cart, but my eyes saw no one. I knew then that the angels of God were there. Was I sorry that I chose to come by handcart? No. Neither then nor any minute of my life since. The price we paid to become acquainted with God was a privilege to pay."[4]

I let this testimony sink in. It had been 395 days of not knowing how I was going to make it through one more day. There were times I didn't know how my body was moving. There were times I didn't know how I survived for the few calories I was consuming. There were times when I didn't know how my body stayed still for the anxiety I felt. There were times when I didn't know how I didn't vomit making dinner for my family. There were countless times I did what I knew I wanted to do as a mother but didn't feel like doing. (Different from just "not wanting" to do something. More like physically incapacitated to do something.) 395 days the Lord not only kept me alive, but blessed me to be there for my family whether or not I was "really there." I didn't do it, He pushed my cart. There is no other explanation.

And so, I stopped fighting. My personal edict to NEVER SURRENDER, *changed*. Changed to COMPLETELY SURRENDER.

Somehow, the gap between what I believed and what is true seemed smaller. And then the healing began. That was almost two months ago. Yesterday I recognized a skip in my step. Last week I thoroughly enjoyed a day at the temple with my husband and children. I can now look ahead more than 12 hours. There is much to heal yet, but it has begun. Perhaps, there is nothing "wrong." Perhaps, it is all "right," for I have become more acquainted with Jesus Christ and His power in my extremities. Isn't that the whole point? **Completely Surrender**. Let Him push your cart.

C H A P T E R

N O T E S

Purpose

1. Jeffrey R. Holland, "Like a Broken Vessel," Ensign, Nov. 2013

2. Julie B. Beck, "What Latter-day Saint Women Do Best: Stand Strong and Immovable," Ensign, Nov. 2007. Quoting Elder John A. Widtsoe in Evidences and Reconciliations, arr. G. Homer Durham, 3 vols. in 1 (1960), 308.

Chapter 2 :: Crisis Period

1. Gordon B. Hinckley, "The Family: A Proclamation to the World," Ensign, Nov. 1995.

Chapter 4 :: Anxiety

1. Erin Holmes, "On Loss and Waiting," BYU Magazine, Winter 2018. Quoting Gregory Clark, "Some Lessons on Faith and Fear," BYU Devotional Address, May 6, 2008.

Chapter 5 :: Infallible Truth, You Are Loved

1. Infallible. (2018) Dictionary.com. Retrieved from www.dictionary.com/browse/infallible?s=t.

2. Dallin H. Oaks, "Powerful Ideas," Ensign, Nov. 1995.

3. Thomas S. Monson, "We Never Walk Alone," Ensign, Nov. 2013.

4. Lynn G. Robbins, "Be 100 Percent Responsible" BYU Devotional Address, August 22, 2017. (IMDb's page for quotes for The Count of Monte Cristo (2002), imdb.com/title/tt0245844/quotes.)

Chapter 7 :: Depression and the Atonement of Jesus Christ

1. Carl B. Cook, "It Is Better to Look Up," Ensign, Nov. 2011.

2. Callister, Tad. The Infinite Atonement. Salt Lake City, Utah: Deseret Book, 2000. p. 124.

3. Ibid, p. 128.

4. Carolyn J. Rasmus, "The Enabling Power of the Atonement," Ensign, March 2014. Quoting David A. Bednar, "In the Strength of the Lord," in Brigham Young University 2001–2002 Speeches (2002).

5. "How Firm a Foundation," LDS Hymns no. 85. Text: Attr. to Robert Keen, ca. 1787. Included in the first LDS hymnbook, 1835. Music: Attr. to J. Ellis, ca. 1889.

6. Redeem. (2018) Dictionary.com. Retrieved from www.dictionary.com/browse/redeem?s=t.

Chapter 8 :: Stigma

1. Stigma. (2018) Dictionary.com. Retrieved from www.dictionary.com/browse/stigma?s=t.

2. Dieter F. Uchtdorf, "Be Not Afraid, Only Believe," Ensign, Nov. 2015.

3. Jeffrey R. Holland, "Like A Broken Vessel," Ensign, Nov. 2013.

4. Stigma. Webster's Seventh New Collegiate Dictionary, 1965.

5. Ibid.

Chapter 9 :: Tender Mercies

1. David A. Bednar, "The Tender Mercies of the Lord," Ensign, May 2005.

Chapter 10 :: Trial of Faith

1. Jeffrey R. Holland, "Like a Broken Vessel," Ensign, Nov. 2013.

2. D. Todd Christofferson, "The Power of Covenants," Ensign, May 2009.

3. Jamie Armstrong, "Michael McLean: You're Not Alone," LDS Living, Nov./Dec. 2016.

4. Neil A. Anderson, "Trial of Your Faith," Ensign, Nov. 2012.

5. Donald L. Hallstrom, "Turn to the Lord," Ensign, May 2010.

6. George Q. Cannon as quoted by Jeffrey R. Holland, "He Hath Filled the Hungry with Good Things," Ensign, Nov. 1997.

Chapter 11 :: Obedience Brings the Blessings of Heaven

1. Russell M. Nelson, "Face the Future with Faith," Ensign, May 2011.

2. David A. Bednar, "Chosen to Bear Testimony in My Name," Ensign, Nov. 2015.

3. M. Joseph Brough, "His Daily Guiding Hand," Ensign, May 2017. Quoting D. Todd Christofferson, "The Power of Covenants," Ensign, May 2009.

Chapter 12 :: You as the "Stewardship"

1. Dieter F. Uchtdorf, "Our Father, Our Mentor," Ensign, June 2016.

2. M. Joseph Brough, "His Daily Guiding Hand," Ensign, May 2017. Quoting Boyd K. Packer, "The Bishop and His Counselors," Ensign, May 1999.

3. Julie B. Beck, "What I Hope My Granddaughters (and Grandsons) Will Understand about Relief Society," Ensign, Nov. 2011.

Chapter 13 :: Prevention is the Best Medicine

1. Jeffrey R. Holland, "Like a Broken Vessel," Ensign, Nov. 2013.

Chapter 14 :: Knowledge is Power

1. "We Thank Thee O God For a Prophet," LDS Hymns, no. 19. Text: William Fowler, 1830–1865, Music: Caroline Sheridan Norton, 1808–ca. 1877.

Chapter 16 : : What Do I Do to Get Healthy?

1. Sarah Knapton, Science Editor, "Depression is a physical illness which could be treated with anti-inflammatory drugs, scientists suggest," The Telegraph, 8 September 2017.

2. Romney, Ann. In This Together: my story. New York: Thomas Dunne Books/St. Martins Griffin, 2015.

3. Lisa Ann Jackson Thomson & Peter B. Gardner, "When the Light Goes Out," BYU Magazine, Spring 2017.

4. Kevin J. Worthen, "It Is Not Good That…Man Should Be Alone," BYU Devotional Address, January 5, 2016.

5. M. Russell Ballard, "The Greatest Generation of Young Adults," Ensign, May 2015.

6. Gregory Clark, "Some Lessons on Faith and Fear," BYU Devotional Address, May 6, 2008.

7. Dieter F. Uchtdorf, "Happiness Your Heritage," Ensign, Nov. 2008.

8. Gordon B. Hinckley, "Put Your Shoulder to the Wheel," New Era, July 2000.

9. Neal A. Maxwell, "Put Your Shoulder to the Wheel," Ensign, May 1998.

10. McConkie, Bruce R., Pathways to Happiness. Salt Lake City: Bookcraft, 1957.

11. Burton, LeVar and Bernardo, Susan Schaefer. The Rhino Who Swallowed a Storm. Burbank, California: Reading Rainbow, 2014.

12. Walch, Tad, "Who is President Russell M. Nelson?" Deseret News, 16 January 2018.

13. Richard G. Scott, "The Transforming Power of Faith and Character," Ensign, November 2010.

HALES

Chapter 17 – Do I Need Therapy?

1. Therapy. (2018) Dictionary.com. Retrieved from www.dictionary.com/browse/therapy?s=t.

2. Sue Bergin, "Real Men Get Help," BYU Magazine, Summer 2016, 21.

3. Pausch, Randy. The Last Lecture. New York, New York: Hyperion Hachette Book Company, 2008.

Chapter 18 – Do I Need Medication?

1. "What Are SSRIs?" WebMD, Retrieved March 15, 2018 from www.webmd.com/depressoin/ssris-myths-and-facts-about-antidepressants#1.

2. For the Strength of Youth. Salt Lake City, Utah: The Church of Jesus Christ of Latter-day Saints, 2001.

Chapter 22 – "Therefore, What?"

1. Orson F. Whitney, in Spencer W. Kimball, Faith Precedes the Miracle (1972), 98.

2. John C. Pingree Jr., "I Have a Work for Thee," Ensign, Nov. 2017.

3. Jeffrey R. Holland and Patricia T. Holland, "Things We Have Learned—Together," Ensign, June 1986.

4. Swinton, Heidi S. To The Rescue, The Biography of Thomas S. Monson. Salt Lake City, Utah: Deseret Book Company, 2010. (Quoting Thomas S. Monson, "Finding Joy in the Journey," 84, 86.)

Epilogue

1. Wendy L. Watson, "Change: It's Always a Possibility!" BYU Devotional Address, April 7, 1998.

2. Lawrence E. Corbridge, "Stand Forever," BYU Devotional Address, January 22, 2019.

3. My Journal, October 16, 2019.

4. David O. McKay, "Pioneer Women," Relief Society Magazine, Jan. 1948, 8.

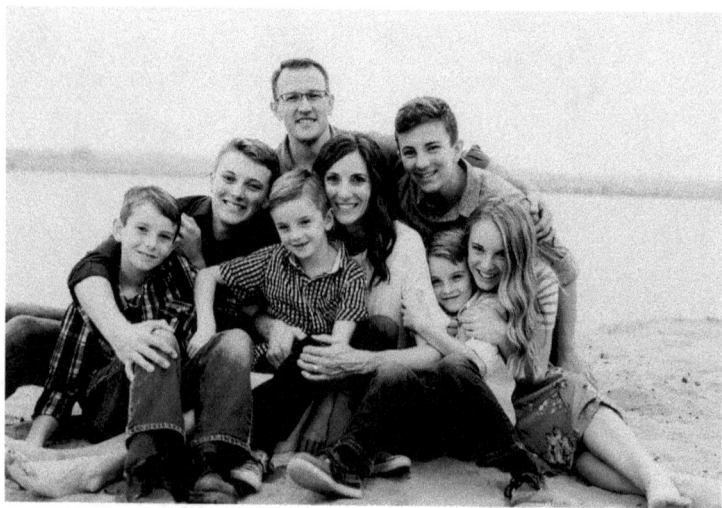

A B O U T   T H E

A U T H O R

Not a stranger to challenges and hard work, Makala grew up a farm girl, the oldest of eight children. Decisively persistent and determined, she was valedictorian of her high school class, a star athlete on a state championship basketball team, and Senior Class President. She graduated at the top of her college nursing class before serving an eighteen-month mission in Ukraine where she daily shared a message about Jesus Christ in Russian. Cultural differences and other challenges like hand-washing her own laundry in a bucket were the norm. Upon her return, she worked as a registered nurse in the Neonatal Intensive Care while completing her bachelor's degree in Marriage, Family, and Human Development at Brigham Young University. She met and married her husband, James, and they welcomed six children into their family, including twin boys as their grand finale. Following the birth of their twins, Makala experienced extreme anxiety and depression which reduced her to a shadow of her former self, sitting in a chair in a darkened corner, unable to cope with the most basic tasks of mothering her young family. She has fought and clawed her way back from those terrible, agonizing depths to regain her former vivacity and happiness, and you can as well! If depression is crushing you, you need to know that there is a way out. It tried to take everything from Makala, but she refused to let it, and she has chosen to take that horrible, dark period of her life and use it to bring light and hope to you, right here, right now.

www.ingramcontent.com/pod-product-compliance
Lightning Source LLC
Chambersburg PA
CBHW071131280326
41935CB00010B/1184